DISEASE
DETECTIVES

DISEASE DETECTIVES

True Stories of NYC Outbreaks

DON WEISS

AVENUE PRESS
MUNN

DISEASE DETECTIVES:
True Stories of NYC Outbreaks
By Don Weiss

First Edition
Copyright © 2025 by Don Weiss
Published by
Munn Avenue Press
300 Main Street, Ste 21
Madison, NJ 07940
MunnAvenuePress.com

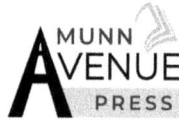

This book is a memoir. It reflects the author's present recollections of experiences over time. Some names and characteristics have been changed, some events have been compressed, and some dialogue has been recreated.

For permission requests, contact MunnAvenuePress.com

Paperback ISBN# 978-1-960299-63-5
Hardcover ISBN# 978-1-960299-81-9

Printed in the United States of America

In memory of Rick, Francisco, Stanley, Irwin, Verne, and Muhammad

Contents

FOREWORD

The detective story is a deeply ingrained part of our culture. But there is another kind of detective who isn't featured in TV shows, despite doing life-saving work. These are the "disease detectives." These epidemiologists and their colleagues work in health departments every day to unravel infectious disease outbreaks and other hazards to protect the public from these usually invisible but potentially life-threatening menaces. The best known of the disease detectives are the officers of the Epidemic Intelligence Service of the CDC (Centers for Disease Control and Prevention), but their counterparts are at work daily solving outbreaks in health agencies all over the world. Like much of public health, this essential work often goes unnoticed.

When these disease detectives get together informally, they reminisce and exchange "war stories," recounting their most instructive or unusual cases. Some of the stories become the stuff of legend, shared with colleagues or passed down through generations of epidemiologists as a sort of oral tradition. Unfortunately, they are rarely written down. This is a pity, because like the more familiar detective stories they are often vivid, suspenseful, and full of surprises.

Luckily for us, with this book Dr. Don Weiss has been addressing this scarcity by giving us a well-chosen selection of iconic cases, making them available at last to the rest of us. These stories make for ripping good yarns and I can't imagine a better guide than Don Weiss. Dr. Weiss is a top infectious disease epidemiologist who has worked for two decades at the New York City Department of Health and Mental Hygiene as Director of Surveillance in the Bureau of Communicable Disease, a prime position for recounting this detective work.

This is also a unique book because it's written by an actual disease detective who can explain the process. One of the author's greatest strengths is his direct personal knowledge of, and often direct involvement in the investigations he describes. The handful of previous books on this topic are mostly written by journalists or science writers. However excellent, they aren't writing from personal experience and may not be aware of some of the details, false leads, and nuances. This book will give you the view from the trenches. With his expertise and personal knowledge, the author demystifies the process to show how field investigations unfold and follows their trail to show what the disease detectives do.

In the process, he artfully weaves in the scientific background and historical context for the general reader. Mention of typhoid fever in New York, of course, brings to mind the famous "Typhoid Mary," a now solved public health mystery of the late 19th and early 20th centuries, but many who read this chapter may well be surprised to learn that typhoid is not just an exotic disease of the past. The background and historical context are effectively interspersed in the narrative, which serves both to inform the reader and build the background for the continuing story.

A central character in the book is New York City itself. The NYC Department of Health and Mental Hygiene is one of the country's largest, with over 5,000 employees and responsibility for over 8 million residents and visitors and has a long history of innovation since its official establishment in 1870. New York City, as a large and diverse urban center at a crossroads of the world, is a prime location for both endemic and emerging infections and has many illuminating public health stories to tell. Weiss is privy to the details of many, and accurately recounts them here, with full credit to the different "shoe leather" epidemiologists who worked on solving these cases, and the teamwork.

Berton Roueché is often considered the originator of the genre of the medical detective story, and perhaps its greatest exponent. Many of these stories, originally published in the *New Yorker* beginning in the 1940's, have become classics and established this genre. With this book, Don Weiss continues the Roueché tradition of explicating fascinating public health mysteries, this time from the vantage point of the investigator.

There is much to learn here, but also much to appreciate – even savor? – as a great story. There are still compelling untold stories, and I hope Dr. Weiss will be giving us more of his tales of the disease detectives.

– Stephen S. Morse, PhD
Professor of Epidemiology
Columbia University Mailman
School of Public Health

CHAPTER 1

Disease Detectives

If one can read their way to writing books, then I got here by reading *Encyclopedia Brown* and science fiction in my formative years. Encyclopedia Brown demonstrated the powers of observation, much like Sherlock Holmes, and how to be an active listener before that phrase entered the lexicon. To embrace science fiction, one had to suspend disbelief and learn science. The stories I read, when not playing ball, aligned with my curiosity about the natural world and enjoyment in finding others' lost items, such as contact lenses or a dongle, retracing their logical fall, bounce, and roll.

Becoming a NYC disease detective (D✪D) wasn't my first job aspiration, or even my first career path. I had started down the road to become a chemist, not the apothecary kind like my uncle, but the bench and Bunsen burner kind. Picture a tweed jacket with leather elbow patches, antique Erlenmeyer flasks lining the shelves of a cluttered office in a small liberal arts college town, surrounded by dairy farms. I wasn't entirely sure that teaching would fulfill the gut-gnawing, deep-held anxiety over what my purpose was, but at least I was going to get educated. I had several good chemistry professor role models: Gerald Roper, who relished beating us whippersnappers in badminton as well as explaining physical chemistry to us; William Schearer, my good-natured college adviser who brought real-world industrial experience to the classroom; and Robert Leyon, the tough, erudite taskmaster, and my first chemistry professor. The chemistry course I enjoyed the most was Advanced Organic Chemistry which required us to identify an unknown substance handed to us in a vial. We'd use standard chemical parameters such as the melting point, solubility, aroma, spectrogram, mass spectroscopy, and nuclear magnetic resonance patterns to make the identification. It was like getting college credit for finding the dean's lost set of keys.

After college, I packed my duffle bag and headed to New Haven for graduate school. "The best laid plans of mice and men oft go awry," is a line from a Robert Burns poem that my first college roommate frequently paraphrased to narrate our freshman gaffes and comes to mind when I think back on those days. I was given a key to Sterling Hall, the chemistry building at Yale University, with the presumption that I would be spending much of the next several years there at all hours of the day and night. But my excitement at owning a key to the castle soon faded. Sterling Hall was built in 1923 in the Gothic style. It was dark, forbidding, and cold. The main hall on the first floor was wide and lit by distant overhead lights that only illuminated the center. One could walk unnoticed, as many grad students did, in the shadows near the walls. I often got lost in the maze of hallways, stairwells, and crevices that at times felt like secret passages to the lairs of mad scientists.

I left Yale after a semester to care for my mother who was dying of cancer. After she died, I stayed at home to give my youngest brother some semblance of stability. I took a job as a synthetic organic chemist making herbicides. One of my coworkers was a middle-aged man who turned out to be a neighbor of a college classmate. He had been with the company for twenty-five years and was stuck because he didn't have an advanced degree. That image frightened me as did the herbicides we produced. Herbicides are chemicals toxic to weeds but less so to crops and people. Poisons nonetheless and chemicals I'm sure Rachel Carlson, author of one of my favorite books, *Silent Spring*, wouldn't have approved. The job wasn't a long-term career path, so I pondered what might come next.

I was not pre-med in college. One episode steered me clear. A classmate in my first-semester biology course didn't do as well on an exam as he had wanted. He returned to his dorm room and proceeded to stab his pillow repeatedly with a knife, or so the story went. True or not there was enough cut-throat behavior among the pre-med cohort to suggest that if this was who I'd have to become to be a physician I needed to find another career.

Chemistry made sense. You could get answers. However, synthesizing noxious compounds became unbearable when I was asked to make a batch of a progenitor compound. The synthesis required phosgene, a gas that was made infamous during WWI as a chemical weapon. While I set up the hood my boss, a PhD chemist, snuck out of the lab to the library claiming he had reading to do. Nonetheless, I made several grams of the foul-smelling, crude-brown gunk, and thought I was done with it. No, the project director ordered me to make two pounds. I asked, if this wasn't the responsibility of the pilot plant? I was given a choice: do the synthesis, quit, or be fired. I resigned and moved on.

I was drawn to medicine for several reasons. Some of my closest friends were in medical school and had shared their positive experiences. I found helping others rewarding and enjoyed solving puzzles. My paternal grandfather had been a physician, so both my parents had hopes that one of their four children would follow in his footsteps. My older brother became a lawyer, and my two younger brothers never met their grandfather. One had his own business and the other became a chemist. The story goes, and this could certainly be a faulty memory, that when I was around three years old, I was observed by my mother playing doctor on a street corner with friends. Twins as I recall. After that I could not convince my mother of any other career possibility.

I attended medical school in Newark, New Jersey. I then trained as a pediatrician in the Bronx and set out to be a community pediatrician. My first jobs were in an urban emergency department and on mobile medical units for homeless children in New York City. Next came working in a federally qualified health center in inner-city St. Louis where the rate of lead poisoning was shockingly high. It prompted me to recall something a colleague said at a conference about changing her career to public health. She was tired of treating society's problems one patient at a time. It made sense to approach disease prevention on a population scale. I returned to school to study epidemiology, an interest stirred by Dr. Donald Louria, a former medical school professor and infectious disease specialist. It took three years of weekend classes to get the degree, and then another three years working in a dysfunctional local public health department before I headed back to my hometown of NYC. That's because, if you wanted a job in public health, NYC's health department was the place to be. After all, NYC is the most densely populated city in the United States and a hub of commerce and travel, there would be no shortage of communicable diseases and mysteries to unravel. I was stepping right into the thick of it when I began working at the department's Bureau of Communicable Diseases (BCD).

The tools of the infectious disease epidemiologist are not

dissimilar from those of the police detective. We both investigate the usual suspects, only ours are microorganisms: such as bacteria, viruses, fungi, and protozoa. While police surveillance involves cameras, ours utilizes data regularly collected on diseases that are reportable by law. Much of the information both disciplines use comes from interviews, be they patients, medical providers, crime victims, or suspects. "Crime" scenes feature in both disciplines, and as will be seen in chapter 6, may overlap. Our crime scenes are often restaurants, congregate facilities, and businesses, as opposed to alleyways and private homes. DNA technology features prominently in both by linking infectious agents with environmental sources as it is used to link crime scene evidence to the suspect.

The Big Apple, Empire City, Gotham, Metropolis. Three hundred square miles dominated by concrete and steel. Home to over eight and a half million people and the daily destination of millions more. The modern incarnation of the department's BCD was created in the 1970s. When I joined in the summer of 2000, BCD was still a small unit of twenty-five but had just witnessed the first of many new age outbreaks: West Nile virus. West Nile virus was unknown in the Western Hemisphere before 1999. Like much of what was to come, it had been imported. Exactly how remains a mystery. Transatlantic crossing or smuggled birds? An infected mosquito in a traveler's luggage? In the bloodstream of a tourist? Regardless, West Nile virus found a home in the Americas and is now with us every summer. A new era of epidemics had begun.

BCD was unlike most units in the NYC Health Department. For starters, we had seventy-three diseases to monitor, investigate, track, and prevent. Literally, from A (Amebiasis) to Z (Zika virus). The Bureaus of Tuberculosis and HIV Prevention and Control each have one disease. The bureaus of Immunization and Sexually

Transmitted Infections have less than ten diseases each. But they all have more staff. Over three-quarters of the BCD staff have specialized training in epidemiology which is the study of disease in populations. At my previous health center job in St. Louis, the similarly prepared proportion was less than a quarter. BCD staff had been pharmacists, teachers, bankers, researchers, pediatricians, and nurses in their former lives, but ultimately became D❂Ds, charged with defending the city from invading microbes. These are our stories.

The stories are presented in nearly chronological order and share a core set of principles and activities. In some instances, patient names and locations have been changed to protect confidentiality. The backbone of infectious disease epidemiology is surveillance, which can be defined as the routine collection, analysis, and dissemination of data on the who, what, where, and when of diseases in humans or animals. The purpose of surveillance is to learn how diseases are acting in a population. The overarching goal of public health is to prevent disease and promote health.

To collect surveillance data, we employ several tools, they include patient or proxy interviews, medical chart reviews, medical provider interviews, site visits, and laboratory testing of people, animals, and the environment. The data is entered into databases and undergoes a variety of analyses including descriptive statistics, calculation of rates, geocoding, mapping, and stratifying by age, sex, geography. Analytical studies are employed to prove or disprove hypotheses on how diseases behave. We use other tools that will appear in some of the stories, but these are the core tools.

Laboratory testing is perhaps the one tool that has changed the most over time. When health departments were first established in the late eighteenth century, and throughout most of the nineteenth century, there were no tests for infectious diseases. In the late nineteenth century, germ theory was accepted, and the new field of microbiology began identifying the causative agents of disease. This was followed by virology in the twentieth century. Diagnostic tests followed each discovery. Ways of growing infectious agents on artificial media or in animal models were perfected. Evidence of human infection or exposure could be detected through culture techniques and markers of immunity—antibodies. The outer surface proteins and lipids of infectious agents are markers that can now be detected with great accuracy. With the elucidation of DNA in the 1950s, a new discipline of molecular epidemiology was soon to be born and has been expanded greatly in the last several decades. Similar to how DNA can be used in forensic criminal investigations to connect a suspect to a crime, DNA, RNA, antibodies, and other proteins associated with infectious agents can be used to solve disease outbreaks.

Three laboratory methods have and continue to play prominent roles in disease investigations. Pulsed-field gel electrophoresis (PFGE) was an early form of "DNA fingerprinting" in which bacteria are grown, their DNA extracted, and then digested with an enzyme that cleaves the molecule in specific locations. It's as if I gave you a piece of string with randomly placed knots and then asked you to cut going left to right before each knot. The digested DNA fragments are then placed on an agarose gel in an electric field that changes direction. The fragments migrate based on their size and charge resulting in a pattern useful when making comparisons. However, PFGE has limited discriminatory power and has largely been replaced by whole genome sequencing (WGS), which allows comparisons of longer DNA sequences. The longer the sequences that can be compared, the greater the certainty there is a match. PFGE and WGS are powerful tools when the question is if the bacteria recovered from a patient is linked to an outbreak or came from an environmental source.

The other laboratory test of great utility to D✪Ds is polymerase chain reaction (PCR). PCR is also based on DNA/RNA technology and is used to determine the presence of an organism in biological or environmental samples. Of note, organisms have unique genetic sequences that, once identified and mapped, can be used to make complementary primers. The primers, DNA polymerase, and the building block nucleotides are placed together in a pool that contains DNA from the organism to be identified. An automated system cycles through various temperatures which allows the primers to combine with the sequence of interest and copy it multiple times. Once sufficiently amplified, the sequence can be detected. This technique is faster than older methods and does not require the organism to be live or viable, just that the specific sequence or sequences are present. So, if there's an envelope with a powder and you wish to be sure it's not anthrax, PCR is the test used.

The authority to conduct public health activities is covered in the Tenth Amendment of the US Constitution, which states that powers not delegated to the United States by the Constitution, nor prohibited by it to the states, are reserved to the states respectively, or to the people. Public health is not mentioned in the Constitution. States, in turn, delegate public health powers to local jurisdictions and cities. New York City's health code delineates the authority of its health department, which includes some that mirror police powers. With an appropriate order by the commissioner of health, a person can be placed in isolation if they are deemed to have an infection that poses a threat to others. This is most often used for tuberculosis control but can occur with other diseases. Quarantine, a term frequently misused by the media, is used when a well person, showing no signs of infection, has been exposed to an infectious agent and is believed to be incubating the disease. Health departments use quarantine sparingly. The goal of isolation and quarantine is to halt transmission of disease. Exclusion is another department power. For example, a child with diarrhea due to salmonella can be excluded from daycare until the illness resolves.

Most of the following chapters are about outbreaks of disease. A few are about a single case. An outbreak is defined as an unusual number of cases of a specific disease in a period of time. This varies by disease and location. A single case of Ebola in NYC, as occurred in 2014, can be considered an outbreak, whereas in parts of Africa, would not. For a disease like salmonella, it's about more than the number of cases. It depends on where, and how the cases are connected.

The steps followed in conducting an outbreak are similar to a recipe. There is an order, but modifications can be made to fit the circumstances. The essential steps are as follows:

1. Establish the presence of an outbreak through surveillance and other data, which includes confirming diagnoses with laboratory tests.
2. Convene an outbreak team and assign responsibilities.
3. Conduct case findings by establishing a case definition and communicating with clinicians and the community.
4. Perform descriptive epidemiology that describes who is at risk by age, sex, geography, and other characteristics.
5. Generate hypotheses about the cause.
6. Conduct special studies such as a case-control study

to evaluate hypotheses, as necessary.

7. Analyze data.
8. Implement control and or prevention measures.
9. Communicate and disseminate findings.
10. Write a report.
11. Continue surveillance to evaluate control measures.

Of note, communication and control measures often come earlier in the sequence and typically require repeating and updating.

Not all D⊗Ds get badges. For the most part, we don't need them to perform our jobs. On a few occasions though, having the assistant commissioner's badge to flash has helped to communicate the seriousness and urgency of a situation.

CHAPTER 2

Guilty Fish

"Can you interview the rabbi's wife?" Sudha asked.

"Sure," I replied. "Is there a questionnaire I should use?"

"No, just see if you can get her to tell you what foods she ate."

It was September 2000. Sudha Reddy was our foodborne disease investigator. She had no dedicated staff so whenever an outbreak occurred, she grabbed whoever was available to help.

The Office of Environmental Investigations, a sister program we worked closely with at the health department, was notified of gastrointestinal illness at six separate events held on September 15 and 16. All six events were catered by the same Manhattan delicatessen. A couple, who had not attended any of the events, but had purchased food from the delicatessen, had also taken ill.

One of the first tasks in any outbreak investigation is to establish a case definition, a set of criteria to identify persons likely to be part of the outbreak. Case definitions typically have several components: symptoms, laboratory tests, time, and place. Time and place are critical to linking the disease to the exposure. For example, when investigating an outbreak at a wedding reception, a person who didn't attend the wedding wouldn't meet the case definition, unless they ate leftovers. Likewise, if the illness was foodborne with symptoms of diarrhea and stomach cramps, a person who had a runny nose after the reception wouldn't meet the case definition either. Getting this right is the basis for trusting the statistics used to implicate a source. The case definition for this outbreak required a person to have diarrhea and at least one other symptom such as stomach cramps, vomiting, or fever. Furthermore, the start of the illness had to be within seventy-two hours of attending one of the events or eating food from the delicatessen. Two of the more critical aspects of foodborne investigations are obtaining leftover food and patient stool specimens. These are necessary to figure out the causative agent, understand the food handling mistake or mistakes that contaminated the food, and link the foods to the human illness; all to take corrective action. Often the illness is short-lived, but people can continue to shed organisms after symptoms end. You'd be surprised how often people are willing to provide stool samples, but it is by no means universal.

I dialed the number for the rabbi's wife. The conversation went something like this:

"Hello?"

Silence.

"Hello? This is Dr. Weiss from the health department."

"My name is Rachel," came the soft reply of a child.

I enjoy speaking with children. They are curious, insightful, and refreshingly honest, that is until they learn how to be deceptive from adults.

"Hi Rachel, is your mother or father home?"

"I'm five years old. I go to kindergarten, but I didn't go today because I'm sick."

"Oh, I'm sorry to hear that. What is wrong with you?"

"I ate guilty fish."

"What?"

"The guilty fish made me sick."

"Oh, when did you eat the guilty fish?"

"I don't know. My fever went away but I still have diarrhea."

"Is anyone else sick?"

"My Nana." I heard the distant voice of an adult followed by a woman's voice asking Rachel to whom she was speaking.

"Hello!? Who 'ist dis?!"

"My name is Dr. Don Weiss. I am calling from the health department."

"Let me tell you about my day. I just finished with the laundry and the dusting. I put my feet up for one minute and what do you know, the telephone rings! I hear Rachel pick up the telephone in the parlor, I hear her telling somebody that she was sick. I thought it was somebody from the school. Oy, I think, I don't need no aggravation!"

"I'm sorry to disturb you. We are investigating a possible episode of food poisoning, and I'd like to ask you some questions."

"Kvestions, always kvestions. You think I stole the crown jewels with all these kvestions. All right, you wanna know what happened at the shul?"

"Is that where the luncheon on September 16th was held?"

"What luncheon? It vas just some knosh after the services."

"Were you in attendance?"

"Women aren't welcomed in the shul."

"So, you didn't eat any of the food?"

"What, I shouldn't eat?"

"So, you did eat the food after the service?"

"Kleyn bisl, a little"

"Ok, I am going to ask you now about each food that was served. Please answer yes or no for each food I mention."

"Are there many people sick?"

"That is what we are trying to find out."

"Did you talk to Mrs. Mandelbaum? She lost her only daughter just last year."

"That's awful, may I continue with my questions?"

"Breast cancer. She vas so young. And with dray little kinder. Oy, such a shame."

"Yes, it is very sad. If I may, did you eat any of the—"

"Mrs. Mandelbaum looks after the kinder, her son is a big shot lawyer."

"—Smoked salmon?"

"I don't care for lox; it gives me heartburn."

"So, you didn't eat any of the smoked salmon."

"I have to watch my cold-less-the-roll."

"Pardon?"

"Cold-less-the-roll. So, my arteries don't harden like my brother Morty."

"What about the lox, did you eat any?"

"What, I shouldn't have? I had a nibble. Was it the lox?"

"What about the kugel?"

"People ate and they enjoyed it!"

"Yes, that's nice, but did you have any of the kugel?"

"I had to see to the kinder. I have two lovely grandchildren. Such joys, Rachel and Aaron."

"Are you saying you left the luncheon early and only ate the smoked salmon?"

"What left? They were only upstairs."

"So, did you eat any kugel?"

"What kugel?"

"The noodle kugel?"

"Yes."

"And the potato kugel?"

"Yes."

"What about the gefilte fish?"

"It vas a nice gefilte fish from the delicatessen. I don't want to speak ill of the dead, but after Harry passed his son-in-law took over the business. He's running it into the ground. That boy don't know stuffed cabbage from borscht. He vas always too busy listening to that rock and rolled music to learn the family business."

"I see, did you eat any of it?"

"I didn't eat much. I am on a diet."

"Are you talking about the gefilte fish?"

"I didn't make it. I told you it vas from the delicatessen. I was too busy with the kinder to make the gefilte. Oy to clean the fish and grind it. It's too much work."

"Yes, I imagine it is. How much of the gefilte fish did you eat?"

"Look, I don't want to get nobody in any trouble. Between you, me and the lamppost, there was something fishy about the gefilte fish, but I don't want no trouble from the government."

"Ma'am, I assure you they won't be in any trouble. We just want to learn what made people sick so we can prevent it from happening next time. Did you eat the gefilte fish?"

"I didn't eat any, it was all gone!"

"Alright. Did you have any cake?"

"My nephew ate the cake."

"He ate the whole cake?"

"Oy, this doctor, such a comedian, you should be on Jerry Seinfeld. He ate some cake. We all ate some cake. It was a good cake. Very moist."

"I just have, hopefully, one more question. Perhaps I should have asked this first. Have you been ill since the sixteenth?"

"I have arthritis."

"Thank you, ma'am. I think that's all I need to know."

A majority of attendees ate all the food, and few responded to our request for an interview—both invalidated statistics used to implicate the foods. It seemed that Rachel was right. The one item served at all events was the gefilte fish. The gefilte fish was prepared in upstate New York, by mixing raw fish (pike, carp, or white fish) with eggs, onion, matzoh meal, and spices. The raw loaves were purchased by the deli and kept frozen. Before sale, the gefilte fish was cooked by boiling in water.

Eleven people submitted stool samples, but a few had mistakenly frozen them. Others were on antibiotics, which can render the culture negative. Still, six people were positive for *Salmonella enteritidis*. No gefilte fish from the events remained and samples obtained from the delicatessen and manufacturer were negative for salmonella. Since eggs can contain salmonella, the batch used was traced back to a farm in Ohio. Samples from the farm were negative for salmonella. The hazard analysis and critical control point (HACCP), a step-by-step review of food preparation and handling, revealed inadequate cooking of the gefilte fish to a sufficient temperature to kill bacteria. An additional violation was the absence of soap and towels at the handwashing station. The two food handlers who prepared the gefilte fish at the delicatessen submitted stool samples and while neither reported eating the gefilte fish or having symptoms, one was positive for *S. enteritidis* and was excluded from work pending follow-up negative stool results. In 2000, molecular analysis of *S. enteritidis* wasn't routine, therefore no comparison of the patient and food handler strains was performed.

Often foodborne investigations don't uncover the smoking gun, or in this case, the putative rotten egg. In this outbreak, there were several plausible explanations. It is still possible that eggs were contaminated with salmonella. and the inadequate cooking of the gefilte fish at the delicatessen allowed the bacteria to multiply. Gefilte fish is served cold, so there would not have been another heating before consumption. Another possibility is that the food handler who tested positive for *S. enteritidis* contaminated the fish during handling. The infectious dose of salmonella is quite high, in the range of 100,000 organisms. For the food handler to have contaminated the exteriors of multiple loaves of gefilte fish to that extent by handling without having symptoms, as reported, seems unlikely. The last possibility is perhaps the most likely: both the food handler and the gefilte fish were contaminated in the delicatessen by environmental bacteria. A study done in 1994 found salmonella on surfaces fifteen inches from a mixing bowl that contained contaminated eggs.[1] Utensils and surfaces remained contaminated after washing and when tested the following day.

There are 1,000 to 1,200 cases of salmonella in NYC every year and this is likely a severe undercount. Most adults who experience diarrhea don't bother to get tested, so they never come to public health's attention. It has been estimated that for every reported case there are fifty that are unreported. Salmonella can survive in the reproductive tracts of hens and therefore can find their way into or onto eggs. The Food and Drug Administration (FDA) does not require that eggs be salmonella-free, only that egg cartons be labeled if the eggs have not been treated in some way to reduce the risk.

Beef and pork are not exempt as the bacteria can live in their gastrointestinal tracts without making the animals ill. During animal slaughter, the bacteria are spread to all parts sold as food. Fruits and vegetables are not risk-free either. Salmonella has been found on strawberries, mangoes, cantaloupes, lettuce, cucumbers, tomatoes, and basil, among others, on raw, washed, and packaged produce. Contamination of crops can occur through the use of natural fertilizers such as manure, irrigation systems, animals, and even humans. The Centers for Disease Control (CDC) estimates that there are over a million salmonella infections in the United States, causing over 25,000 hospitalizations, and more than 400 deaths annually. Fifteen multistate outbreaks caused by salmonella have occurred in the United States in the first seven months of 2024, and these are just the ones that have been detected and investigated by the CDC.[2]

During my time with the health department, we did about fifty foodborne investigations per year. There were small local outbreaks associated with a specific eatery and large multistate ones linked to a commercial product. There were those in which the outbreak was detected by a cluster of case reports and others where illness was reported but no organism was ever identified. Weddings, catered corporate events, and graduation ceremonies were common outbreak venues, but foodborne illness occurs most often on a smaller scale. A group of friends dine together at a restaurant, share food, and then become ill. After unpacking on the day I moved back to NYC in 2000, I visited a neighborhood specialty foods store choosing a package of store made crab cakes for dinner. The day after eating the crab cakes I developed food poisoning. Perhaps the universe was sending the message that if I was going to do this work for the next two decades, I ought to know how the victims of disease felt.

Reducing the quantity of salmonella entering the food chain is one component of control, however, it is unrealistic to believe we can reach a zero level. Individuals can protect themselves and others by hand washing after handling poultry, meat, and eggs and avoiding cross-contamination of potential salmonella-containing foods with uncooked foods such as salads. Wash fruits and vegetables. Heat kills salmonella, so cook eggs and meat thoroughly.

CHAPTER 3

Typhoid Chicken

I was sitting in my office early one morning in December 2010 when José rushed in very excited. There weren't many staff around yet and the expression he wore was of someone looking to celebrate a success. José was a public health epidemiologist (PHE) with fifteen years of experience investigating cases for the bureau. He was waving a lab report around in the air, pumping a fist, and smiling. He then repeated, "I got her! I got her! It was the babysitter!" I managed to calm him down long enough to explain.

A few weeks earlier José was assigned a typhoid fever (TF) case in a four-year-old child. The first step of a TF investigation is to establish a history of travel. Thirty-five percent of New Yorkers are foreign-born and journey to their native countries to visit friends or family. Often, they return to the United States with more than photos and memories. The CDC estimates that there are over 9 million cases of TF each year worldwide.[3] While New Yorkers comprise 3% of the US population, they make up 15% of the nation's annual TF fever burden.

José had quickly learned that the family had not traveled recently and all family members other than the child had tested negative. Both parents worked and the child did not attend daycare. That meant there had to be another childcare arrangement. José tracked down the babysitter and it took more than a week to arrange for her stool to be tested, a frequent problem in TF investigations. While we humans have no qualms about picking up our dog's poop, we are reluctant to provide our excrement for analysis. The lab report José was waving revealed that the forty-two-year-old babysitter had typhoid bacilli in her stool. We suspected she was a carrier, like Typhoid Mary, and had passed the infection to the four-year-old. José's case reminded me of an outbreak we investigated in my first year as a D✪D.

Typhoid fever is caused by *Salmonella typhi*, a member of the salmonella family of bacteria, and a disease that only affects humans. It is transmitted by hands, food, or water contaminated by feces and it usually requires an inoculum of 100,000 or more organisms to get past the killing effect of stomach acid. However, some strains are capable of infecting with as few as ten bacteria. Illness usually occurs one to two weeks after ingestion but may be as long as sixty days later depending on the quantity of bacteria ingested, host, and strain factors.

Once the bacteria reach the small intestine, they can penetrate the intestinal wall. White blood cells then swallow them up but are unable to destroy the invaders. The bacteria multiply and enter the bloodstream. If untreated 10–20% of those affected will die. After surviving, 1–4% of TF cases become chronic carriers; people with no apparent symptoms who intermittently shed the bacteria in their stool and can transmit the disease to unsuspecting others through poor personal hygiene.

The responsibility for monitoring TF in New York City belonged to Sudha Reddy. When Sudha joined the D✪Ds in December of 1999 she was a twenty-seven-year-old epidemiologist who had spent nearly her whole life in Georgia. After completing her graduate studies at Emory University's Rollins School of Public Health she spent three years with the FoodNet Program at the CDC. Her work at the CDC consisted of data analysis and phone consultation with local health departments. Sudha wasn't looking for a new job, but when the opportunity arose to work in NYC, she couldn't resist the lure of life in a big city and epidemiology on the front lines. She arrived in NYC in the dead of winter, and being accustomed to mild Georgia winters, rarely emerged from her apartment until the spring thaw.

The summer of 2000 kept Sudha busy. People spend time outdoors grilling and consuming barely refrigerated food. In addition to the outbreak of *Salmonella enteritidis* in the delicatessen-prepared gefilte fish, there was an outbreak at a hospital luncheon due to enterotoxin *Escherichia coli*, and on Labor Day, a cruise ship party took ill with *Vibrio parahaemolyticus*. The PHEs were busy too. In August there were seven cases of TF. Staff discovered that four of them had traveled to endemic countries Guatemala, Nigeria, and Bangladesh, however, three did not report travel nor another exposure.

Most NYC TF cases are related to travel. When you added up the proportion that traveled, consumed imported food, had contact with a recent traveler to an endemic country, or lived in a house with a carrier, only 6% of cases remained unexplained. Experience taught us that these individuals either had reasons to deny travel or contact with a traveler. Distrust of government, tenuous immigration status, or unauthorized leave are the chief reasons people keep mum on their whereabouts. But occasionally a case didn't realize that they had consumed imported food. Mexico was the most common travel destination of TF cases, but a significant number had gone to Bangladesh, India, and Pakistan. Nearly all the TF cases initially thought to be non-travel were eventually linked to an infectious carrier in the home.

The protocol for TF investigations was well-worn. Upon receipt, the report is entered into the surveillance database and the face sheet printout is given to the borough PHE supervisor for assignment. A copy of the report is then given to Sudha. The PHE conducts an investigation that includes interviewing the patient and a chart review if the patient is hospitalized. If the patient did not report any of the usual risk factors, such as travel, the PHE would immediately notify Sudha. These are merely the first steps of the investigation. Household contacts of the case had to be screened for occupation and typhoid status. To prevent outbreaks, food handlers, day care, and health care workers exposed to a case of TF are excluded from work until three stools are negative for *S. typhi*. This means collecting stool specimens. The patient is followed for three months after the completion of antibiotic therapy, if used, to identify individuals shedding the organism. If they are in a high-risk profession they too cannot return to work until cleared. It's burdensome for families as well as D✪Ds, but necessary to prevent a return of the deadly disease.

TF thrives wherever sanitation is poor. Before modern sewer systems, TF was an urban scourge affecting an estimated 1 of every 1,000 residents. That might not seem like much but consider that in 2018 that figure had dropped to 1 in 88,000 persons.[4] During the Civil War it is estimated that over 75,000 soldiers contracted TF and more than 25,000 perished.[5] The largest outbreak in the United States in recent years occurred in a migrant camp in Florida in 1973 where 210 persons took ill.[6] The source of TF transmission is typically from a carrier, like the infamous NYC cook Mary Mallon, or contaminated water. But sources from snow cones to watermelon have been implicated in outbreaks.[7]

Although the details unfolded over several weeks, Sudha

realized we had a TF outbreak when six case reports were received over six days. On Thursday, September 28, 2000, the first two TF reports came from different hospitals and were assigned to the Queens field team. It wasn't unusual to receive two cases from Queens as historically about 40% of TF cases came from the borough (county), which is the most ethnically diverse of the five NYC boroughs. The next day, a physician from a Manhattan hospital called to report two more TF cases, including that neither had traveled. Both patients were young women and residents of Queens. The following Tuesday, October 3, two more TF cases without travel were reported—one from Queens, the other from Manhattan.

Six TF cases in such a short interval was unusual. In the previous twenty-five years, there had been only one outbreak of non-travel-associated TF in NYC. In 1990, seven cases in Northern Manhattan were traced to a baptism luncheon.[8] Dr. Tom Frieden, who twenty-two years later would become NYC health commissioner, performed the investigation. It turned out that the cook who made the potato salad was a carrier. Through negligent hygiene, she had contaminated food that was not heated before consumption—like the gefilte fish outbreak.

In 2000, BCD was a small bureau. With three nurse epidemiologists, nine field investigators, two research scientists, four physicians, and three administrative staff, we fit neatly into three rooms on the third floor of 125 Worth Street in Lower Manhattan. Four of the field investigators were dedicated to waterborne parasitic diseases, which left five field investigators to cover sixty-plus diseases occurring in over 8 million people. The Queens field team was overwhelmed, to say the least. It was imperative to confirm the absence of travel and begin looking for other exposures so that further transmission could be prevented. TF investigations are complicated by the fact that, in terms of enteric diseases, the disease has an average incubation period of weeks instead of days. People have a hard enough time recalling where they had been and what they ate in the past two days let alone during the previous two weeks.

While the field team focused on chart reviews, Sudha put aside her other outbreak work and mapped the six cases by home address. Three cases came from the same Central Queens neighborhood—one from an adjacent neighborhood and one from the next neighborhood to the west. The lone case outside of Queens lived in the Lower East Side of Manhattan, coincidentally the same neighborhood Sudha had moved to just a month earlier. Sudha next began making calls to re-interview the patients.

Luis was a twenty-two-year-old man originally from Central America and the first case of the cluster reported. He became ill on September 20 with fever and body aches. He was hospitalized four days later with *S. typhi* bacilli in his blood. Luis had moved to the States as a child, was the only male of the cluster, and worked in a repair shop. It took a week to reach him for an interview. Sudha learned that he had not traveled in the month before getting sick, however, he received a visitor from his homeland who brought bread and candy that he ate. None of his roommates were ill but as per protocol, they were asked to submit stool specimens. Luis could not recall the names of restaurants he ate at during the month before the illness.

Sudha next contacted Olivia, a thirty-three-year-old woman who had fever and nausea beginning on September 18. On the fifth day of her illness, she was seen in a Queens hospital where blood tests were drawn, and she was sent home. Two days later the blood test confirmed TF, she was recalled and admitted for antibiotic therapy. Olivia was born in South America and worked in non-clinical health care. Her elderly parents lived with her and were reported to be well with no history of TF. She denied contact with foreign travelers or imported food and had traveled only to Florida. Olivia's recall of the restaurants she patronized in the month before her illness, now nearly two months ago, was excellent. She listed eight, seven of which were in Queens, the other in Manhattan; she even recalled the foods eaten at each location. This was a huge clue.

The third case interviewed that first week of October was a thirty-three-year-old woman named Darlene who was born in the Dominican Republic but had resided in NYC since the age of three. Her illness began on September 20 with a fever of 103.9 °F, vomiting, diarrhea, and abdominal pain. After five days of symptoms, Darlene visited a Manhattan hospital where she was admitted and two days later the diagnosis of TF was made. She was self-employed and didn't eat out, a rarity for a New Yorker. Darlene was the outlier because of her Manhattan residence and her absence of restaurant exposure. As a result, Darlene's presence in the cluster raised the possibility of a contaminated commercial product being distributed beyond Queens.

Samantha, the fourth case, took ill with a headache and a temperature of 103°F on September 18. The oldest of the six cases at a mere thirty-five years, Samantha worked in Manhattan in finance and lived with her parents in Queens. Her headache was so severe and accompanied by a stiff neck that when she arrived at the emergency department the physicians evaluated her for meningitis and performed a CT scan and spinal tap. In her blood was where they found the offending *S. typhi bacilli*. She too had none of the traditional risk factors for TF and her recall of restaurants equaled that of Olivia, recalling eleven establishments.

By the fourth day of October, four of the six cases had

been interviewed. Sudha paused to review their questionnaire responses for common themes, but several things already stood out. All four cases were young adults who had onset of illness on either September 18 or 20. Incubation periods, the time from exposure to the start of symptoms, can be a clue and depend on the dose of the infecting agent, strain, and host factors. In general, the longer the mean incubation period of a pathogen the wider the range in values one expects for a series of cases, even those exposed around the same time. For a disease like TF with a mean incubation period of two weeks, it was unusual to see such clustering of onsets. It strongly suggested that all the cases were exposed during a narrow window of time and with a similar dose of bacteria. This pattern would be rare for a commercial product contamination as people purchase and consume store-bought foods over a wide range of time. It suggested to Sudha a point source: It had to be a restaurant.

Luis hadn't been able to recall where he ate out in August, so Sudha arranged for him to be reinterviewed in his native Spanish. Darlene confided that she was on a restricted weight loss diet so rarely ate out. Olivia and Samantha both listed the same restaurant in Queens called Malpolrica. Sudha knew it often took several interviews before cases recalled places where they ate. Maybe they'd find a receipt or ask a friend. Memory was also improved if investigators used a prepared list, analogous to a victim viewing a police lineup of suspects through a one-way mirror. From the restaurants named by Olivia and Samantha, Sudha removed restaurants not in Queens and created a lineup list to be incorporated into a supplemental questionnaire. Sudha also called Faina, the supervisor of the department's restaurant inspection unit, and requested that an inspector be sent post-haste to Malpolrica.

While Sudha was busy preparing a new questionnaire, two

more non-travel-associated TF cases were reported. One was a ten-year-old boy from Queens and the other a five-year-old boy from Brooklyn. Their ages didn't fit the pattern, and Sudha couldn't imagine how the five-year-old from Brooklyn could be exposed to an eatery on a side street in Queens. Interviews and screening tests led to the discovery that he was exposed to his grandmother who was a carrier. The ten-year-old had no connection to Malpolrica or any other explanation for his infection and would have to await the molecular typing results to see if he was part of the burgeoning outbreak.

At the time, determining whether *S. typhi* strains were linked to each other, a carrier, or a common source, utilized PFGE. In PFGE, bacterial DNA is split into pieces and the patterns created when the fragments migrate through a gel under the influence of an electric field are compared by a computer program. It is not as specific as fingerprinting is for solving crimes, but for many organisms, it is an indispensable tool in outbreak investigations. If two bacterial PFGE patterns have the same number and position of bands on the gel, we say that the two strains are indistinguishable. PFGE isn't perfect, it lacks the discriminatory power of more advanced genetic analyses, but it was the best available tool at the time. Results generally took one to two weeks and were not yet available that first week of October 2000.

The inspection of Malpolrica took place on October 5. Several violations were noted, the worst being bare hand contact with food and inadequate holding temperatures. The inspector witnessed a cook placing tomato slices as garnishes on plates without gloved hands and spotted two pots of prepared meat sitting next to the stove. When a thermometer was inserted into the pots it read 97°F instead of the required 140°F or greater. The bare hands of an unsanitary carrier could introduce *S. typhi bacilli* and cooling food is a setup for bacterial multiplication. The inspector also noted that the handwashing sink did not have soap.

Malpolrica employed eleven people including the two owners. All food handlers were given stool specimen kits and told that they would be excluded from work if they did not comply. All the employees complied, except one—Marcos, the delivery person. He reportedly didn't prepare food and we were told that he had left his job several weeks earlier.

Armed with the new questionnaire, Sudha returned to calling the cases. Two had yet to be reached for the initial interview and the rest needed to be reinterviewed using the new restaurant list. Sudha next spoke with Missy, a twenty-year-old woman whose illness began before the other cases. Her fever started on September 16 and peaked at 104°F. The fever was accompanied by malaise, chills, vomiting, and abdominal pain. Like Olivia, she visited an emergency department where she was examined, and blood was drawn. She was advised to take antipyretics and released. Two days later the hospital called. She needed to return immediately to be treated for TF. Missy lived in Queens but attended university in Manhattan. The case count had reached eight: five cases lived in Queens, but three now had a connection to Manhattan.

Sudha methodically administered the new questionnaire to Missy eliminating travel, contact with a carrier or a recent traveler to a typhoid-endemic country, and consumption of imported foods as risk factors. Other than seeing her father, who had returned from a trip to Hong Kong where TF is not endemic, all her answers were no. The first restaurant on the list was a sandwich shop chain and Missy recalled eating at, but a different branch than the other patient. Two more were familiar as places she ate, including Malpolrica.

Sophia's story was much the same. She took ill on September

18 with fever, headache, and chills. She then visited the emergency department of a Queens hospital where she was told that it was probably the flu and to go home, rest, and drink fluids. But Sophia's fever persisted and on September 26 she returned to the emergency department and was hospitalized. Two days later her blood culture was positive for *S. typhi*. Born in the Dominican Republic and living in the United States since a teenager, the twenty-two-year-old worked in an office and denied travel or eating imported foods. She lived in Queens with three roommates and recalled receiving visitors from Puerto Rico in the first week of September, none of whom were ill. One of her roommates did have a diarrheal illness in July and was evaluated by a physician but was never tested for TF. When Sudha read off the restaurant list, Sophia reported eating at a sandwich shop, but not the one on the list. She also ate at the pizza restaurant and had takeout from one other restaurant—Malpolrica. What's more, on four Sundays in August she ate their steak, empanadas, and rice and beans. The evidence was lining up.

On October 12, Sudha took a breath to review her notes and summarize the findings. Four of the six cases ate at the same Queens restaurant, Malpolrica. Darlene didn't fit the pattern as she lived in Manhattan and denied visits to all the restaurants on the list. Although the cases didn't report eating the same food at Malpolrica, there was little doubt in Sudha's mind that Malpolrica was involved in the outbreak. But was it the only source location? Food handlers sometimes work at multiple restaurants and change jobs frequently. The Manhattan outlier also raised the possibility that a contaminated commercial or restaurant product could be involved and in use by other restaurants in the city. Sudha also knew of an outbreak of TF that occurred in Florida in 1999 that was caused by imported frozen mamey concentrate used to make fruit shakes.[9] Darlene's illness troubled Sudha. While she fit the patient profile of being a young woman with onset in mid-September, she swore that she hadn't visited Queens. It would be another week before the results of the PFGE analysis would reveal which cases were linked, but there was something Sudha considered doing in the meantime.

The morning of Friday, October 13, was bright and sunny. Sudha verified Darlene's address. It was a few blocks north and east of her apartment, close to the East River in a cluster of high-rise buildings named for the famous Dutch photographer, Jacob Riis. Sudha figured it would be unlikely to find Darlene home at 9:30 a.m. but she decided to give it a try anyway. She located her building and slipped through the security door as someone exited. Sudha took the elevator to the twelfth floor and knocked on apartment D. A petite woman with dark hair opened the door. Sudha introduced herself and was invited inside.

After explaining the nature of her visit and the status of the investigation, Sudha pulled from her bag the questionnaire. She started by confirming the details of Darlene's illness previously obtained by phone interview and chart review. Sudha asked again about travel. Some TF cases upon persistent questioning eventually confide that they had indeed traveled internationally. Darlene had not traveled. She had no contact with foreign visitors or friends who had recently traveled. She told Sudha that she was self-employed and made jewelry. She frequently traveled to New Jersey to attend craft fairs and flea markets. She also stated that she had not been to Queens during the past year. She confirmed that she did not eat at Malpolrica nor at any of the restaurants on the list. Darlene explained that to control her weight she made most of her food, favoring salads and cooked vegetables over processed foods. In addition, she had recently been through a detoxification program and was following the guidance of a nutritionist. There was something about the way she discussed her weight that made Sudha suspect there was more to the story. She listened attentively. Darlene bought all of her groceries at a local supermarket and ate chicken or fish about once per week. There was one exception. While in Yonkers in mid-September she stopped at a diner on Central Avenue and ate a turkey burger.

Darlene lived alone and sometimes visited her family in the Bronx. Sudha saw an opening and felt she had established sufficient rapport to broach the delicate subject. TF was occasionally transmitted by sex partners. Did Darlene have a boyfriend? No, she didn't, well, she used to. The breakup was months ago but it was still raw. She began to cry. Sudha consoled her as only a young woman herself, alone in NYC, could. The meeting ended without determining how Darlene had become infected. Sudha thanked her for her time and left a number she could call in the event she remembered anything.

Early the following Monday morning, Dr. Jim Rahal, an infectious disease physician from Queens, called our assistant commissioner, Marci Layton. He reported three cases of non-travel TF at his hospital and as they all lived in Queens, he wanted to make sure we were aware and investigating a possible cluster. One of the cases we were aware of but the other two were new. Their onsets were in mid-September like the others, so it didn't necessarily mean that exposure was ongoing. But we prioritized the cases for interviews anyway.

Kiki was a college student from Queens studying to become a nurse. The nineteen-year-old moved to the United States from Hong Kong at age seven and recalled a brief illness on September 4 that she thought could have been the flu. A week and a half later, the fever returned, and her private physician treated her with antibiotics for a urinary tract infection. She stopped taking the antibiotics when the urine culture returned negative. Less than a week later, Kiki was again ill, but this time the fever climbed to 105°F. On October 8, she was admitted to a Queens hospital and TF was diagnosed a few days later. Kiki recalled eating plantains, rice and beans, and perhaps some chicken at Malpolrica with a friend on September 11. She had no other risks for TF.

Twenty-four-year-old Roberta moved to NYC from Western Europe and was also attending college. Her illness began on September 17 and featured intermittent fever of 105°F, headaches, night sweats, chills, diarrhea, and abdominal pain. During her second visit to the same hospital as Kiki on October 12, she was admitted for antibiotic treatment. It was soon discovered that she too had TF. Other than contact with her husband, who had traveled to the Middle East but was vaccinated against TF, Roberta had none of the traditional risk factors. She had eaten at several locations, including her college cafeteria, street vendors, and a wedding reception. It came as little surprise when she recognized Malpolrica on the list of restaurants.

October 2000 was my fourth month as a D✪D. My assignments had mostly been writing protocols and devising ways to improve our surveillance system. My experience with foodborne outbreaks had been limited. In the gefilte fish outbreak, my role was confined to a difficult interview that didn't add much to the investigation, so I was more than ready for an investigation I could sink my teeth into.

Sudha was at her desk preparing a medical alert to send to hospitals and physicians about the outbreak when a call for her came into the office front desk. It was Darlene. She remembered something from the summer, a place in Queens where she spent several afternoons and nights. The place was called Tickles and was an exotic dancer nightclub. While Darlene talked Sudha looked up the address, it was less than a mile from Malpolrica. Darlene explained that she went there to sell jewelry one night and ended up befriending the dancers becoming a sort of mother hen. Darlene sold a few items, did makeup, and doled out boyfriend advice. She believed that Malpolrica was the place the girls ordered food from. Darlene thought that she had a fruit drink and maybe took a bite of someone's chicken while she was at Tickles.

Every Tuesday the bureau holds a staff meeting to discuss new cases and outbreaks and review the status of ongoing ones. Sudha presented the non-travel TF investigation on October 17. There were nine unexplained cases in less than four weeks and all but one were adults. With Darlene's recollection, there were now five cases who reported eating at Malpolrica, one who didn't, and three who still needed to be reinterviewed. All but two of the nine cases lived in Queens, and except for the ten-year-old boy, the age range was very narrow—nineteen to thirty-five. Laura at the Public Health Lab (PHL) set up the PFGE gel and results were expected before the week's end.

After the outbreak meeting, a tenth non-travel TF was reported. When we reached the doctor who cared for the thirty-seven-year-old woman we learned that her onset was on October 8, beyond the current window of the other cases. Because of the long and variable incubation period of TF, it was still possible that she was infected by an exposure in late August or early September, but it raised the very real concern that transmission was ongoing. The woman lived in Queens but in a section removed from the other cases and the restaurant. However, she worked within a few blocks of Malpolrica. She couldn't recall the name of the restaurant but admitted ordering takeout several times a week before her illness from a place she described as serving Spanish food and matching the street coordinates of Malpolrica. The one wrinkle was that she named another restaurant, a Chinese food place, that another TF patient had also mentioned during her interview. It could be a coincidence, but it raised a dollop of doubt.

At about 2:30 p.m. on October 17, Marci called Sudha and me to her office to discuss the outbreak. We decided to make a surprise visit to the restaurant. I had completed the paperwork to become an approved department driver, so we grabbed a car and sped out to Queens accompanied by a Spanish-speaking restaurant inspector. It was nearly 5:00 p.m. when we arrived. It was a congested section of Queens, on a wide boulevard with a mall. We located Malpolrica off the main boulevard. It was small, the dining area no more than 300 square feet, yet was filled with about a dozen square, white tables, about half of which were occupied. The walls were brightly painted, and the place appeared clean. Three employees served food from a walk-up window behind which was a closet-sized kitchen. The menu was extensive considering the size of the kitchen—eggs, soups, an array of appetizers, chicken, pork, steak, and seafood could be had—most for under $12. One could order takeout for several months and not eat the same meal twice.

We met Carmen, the forty-ish co-owner, and explained the purpose of our visit. We commandeered a couple of tables in the back that weren't any more private than a subway car to conduct staff interviews. We each took a separate table and questioned the eight employees who were present; one was said to be on vacation. Senator Joseph McCarthy conducted his purge of Communism before I was born, but I imagined the interrogations must have felt similar for his quarry as they did for the employees. We asked about illness, specifically if any were ever told they had TF. For most English was not their first language, and though I spoke a little Spanish, I couldn't be sure our questions were fully understood. The one word in English they all knew though was no. No illness. No travel. No imported food. No contact with someone with diarrhea. One woman I interviewed made a habit of answering my questions before the words had left my mouth.

I moved to the counter where Carmen was busy with phone calls and packaging takeout orders. The place was much busier than I had expected as it was not quite dinner time. I then asked her about Marcos, her phantom deliveryman. She told me she didn't know his address. While I found that hard to believe I tried not to let it show. Did Marcos ever handle food? She told me no, that he was full-time on deliveries. Where was he from? Was anyone here a friend of his? Did he give an emergency contact or a place to send his final paycheck? Carmen didn't know. I told her we planned a return visit to draw blood from everyone and that the tests would show us if anyone was a carrier. Expecting indifference, I noted that her attention briefly drifted away from tossing plastic forks in the takeout orders before she bid me a good day. On the way out of the restaurant, I asked the waiter to take me to the basement. There was a narrow refrigerator with a glass door, the kind often containing soft drinks in a bodega. On the bottom shelf was a bag of frozen mango and a pitcher of a premixed shake.

The next day, October 18, we received the first batch of PFGE reports. Six of the cases were analyzed and five, including Darlene, were indistinguishable. The other differed by a single band meaning that it was very likely all six cases were infected by the same source. We suspected the remaining three cases would match the outbreak strain too when the next PFGE batch was run. The isolate from the ten-year-old boy from Queens wasn't part of the run so we'd have to wait several more weeks to learn if he was part of the outbreak.

Sudha did what she could to locate Marcos. She looked him up in our surveillance database to see if he was a known case or carrier of TF. No luck. She used our subscription database of addresses and phone numbers, but he wasn't listed. It was not uncommon for several food handlers in NYC to live together in a one-bedroom apartment with only a cell phone, so unless he turned himself in we weren't going to find him, that is if he even existed. I had my doubts. The list of employees we received from Malpolrica's accountant oddly didn't include anyone named Marcos. We were told he was paid off the books.

We returned to Malpolrica the following week armed with phlebotomy equipment. Stool samples on the food handlers were thus far negative, which can happen with intermittent shedders of *Typhi bacilli*, that's why we required three samples separated by days before concluding the person was negative. The CDC had developed a blood test for the virulence capsular polysaccharide (Vi) antibody that helped identify TF carriers. A person who has *S. typhi* in their system, but shows no signs of illness, has established a sort of détente with the bacterium. The immune system of a carrier can prevent the overt symptoms of fever and diarrhea but cannot eradicate the organism completely. The truce is due to the Vi antibody, named for a surface protein of *S. typhi*. We drew blood on all the food handlers and asked again about illness, emphasizing that a bout of TF could have occurred anytime in their life. We were again told no. The Vi antibody test results would take a week. From the freezer downstairs we collected unopened bags of frozen papaya, passion fruit, and mango concentrate for testing.

The next few weeks were relatively uneventful. There were two more non-travel TF cases; a fifty-two-year-old woman from

Manhattan and a thirty-two-year-old woman from Brooklyn. Neither were linked to the restaurant. The second PFGE analysis revealed that the ten-year-old boy did not match the outbreak strain, but the isolates from Kiki, Roberta, and Missy did. Repeat case interviews raised the total who reported eating at Malpolrica to eight with the lone unlinked case not yet interviewed a second time. Two stool samples from each of the ten food handlers were all negative. And we had yet to find Marcos.

The CDC laboratory in Atlanta called Sudha on November 2 with the results of the Vi antibody tests. All the waiters and cooks were negative. Carmen, the co-owner, was positive. CDC was confident of the results, and it suggested, despite her having a pair of negative stools, that she was a chronic typhoid carrier. It looked like the case was solved. We decided to ask Carmen to come to our offices to go over the results and explain what would happen next.

We borrowed the office of the commissioner's chief of staff to meet with Carmen, it presented a nicer face of the health department than either of our cubicles or even Marci's office which was overcrowded and had a window that faced a roof of exhaust fans. After explaining the test results to her we again inquired about her medical history. She recalled childhood illnesses in her native country of Colombia, but we couldn't say for sure that it was TF. She had also never been tested or told she was a carrier. Carmen again insisted that she didn't handle food at the restaurant. Aside from the administrative work, she took phone calls or worked the register. Sudha pressed her. What about when someone calls in sick or fails to show up for work? That never happens was her reply. We recalled our visit during off hours and how busy it was. We asked Carmen if it was possible that during the lunch or dinner rush she handled food? Under the warmth of Sudha's non-threatening quizzical look, Carmen finally admitted that on rare occasions she helped with food preparation, but she was always careful to wash her hands.

Carmen was excluded from the restaurant and was ordered to submit three additional stool specimens per week for four weeks before we agreed to reinstate her. The first two specimens would be obtained by rectal swab at a department clinic that treats sexually transmitted diseases. A bit Draconian, but we needed to ensure the chain of custody. We worried she might submit another person's stools if she suspected, as we did, that she was the source of the outbreak. If any of the tests were positive she had two treatment options. One involved a four-week course of antibiotics and the other an evaluation of and possible surgery to remove her gallbladder, the favorite hiding place of *S. typhi* bacteria. If the first option failed the second would be considered.

A month later, with no new cases linking to Malpolrica, we got the final stool results. No typhoid was recovered from any of Carmen's stool specimens. We did not request urine samples but in retrospect perhaps this was an oversight as some carriers excrete only through the urine. Carmen was allowed to return to work and a repeat surprise restaurant inspection was scheduled while we kept a cautious eye out for additional cases.

In 1907 the field of bacteriology was in its infancy. It was the case of Typhoid Mary that first brought the concept of healthy typhoid carriers to light in the United States. Most people have heard of Typhoid Mary, if not her real-life story, then at least comprehend how the moniker applies to putative carriers of disease. Over several years, twenty-two cases of TF occurred in seven different homes where Mary Mallon was employed as a cook. When investigator George Soper turned this information over to the NYC Health Department an inspector visited Mary Mallon to question her. Mary's refusal to cooperate led to her forcible removal and detention on North Brother Island. Two years later she had her day in court but the New York Supreme Court judge who heard the case refused to set her free, upholding the health department's right to infringe on individual civil rights to protect public health. Mary was eventually released with a promise not to cook and to report to the health department for regular examinations. She did neither and was recaptured five years later after another TF outbreak at her place of employment. Mary Mallon was sent back to North Brother Island for the remainder of her life.[10]

As we pondered what options we had to prevent further cases of TF associated with Malpolrica, the specter of Mary Mallon haunted our hallways. The evidence against Mary Mallon was both epidemiologic and bacteriologic. From her feces on repeated occasions was cultured *S. typhi*. Despite the inexperience with such microbiologic evidence at the time her incarceration was upheld.

The evidence suggesting that Carmen was a typhoid carrier, and responsible for the outbreak, was similar to the Mallon case. The same two categories of evidence tied her to the nine TF cases, however, the epidemiology linking Carmen to the cases in 2000 was not as strong as with Mary Mallon. The Vi antibody was a blood marker suggestive of a carrier state, not evidence that the causative bacteria was still in her system. Our pursuit of the Malpolrica typhoid carrier ended when cases stopped, and no typhoid was recovered from the frozen fruit packages. The restaurant was never closed, and no civil liberties were infringed.

A year following the outbreak, in the aftermath of 9/11 and in the middle of the anthrax letters investigation, there was another cluster of non-travel TF. Three men were diagnosed with TF;

two of them were residents of Queens who had indistinguishable PFGE patterns to the strain found in the Malpolrica restaurant cluster. None of the men recalled eating at the restaurant and harried staff quickly moved on to more pressing tasks. Thankfully, the strain has not shown up again in the years since.

Meanwhile, José was wrapped up in the 2010 TF case connected to the babysitter. The woman's *S. typhi* isolate matched by PFGE to the child and she was treated with antibiotics for four weeks. Follow-up stool tests all tested negative. It looked like she had been cured of her carrier state. I thought about Malpolrica and felt a bit like Inspector Morell in *The Girl with the Dragon Tattoo*. I had left something unresolved.

Ten years had passed with no new cases and memories faded like Polaroid snapshots. The Malporica *S. typhi* outbreak PFGE pattern was stored in a database at the CDC and had been described as a rare strain. The author of that assessment still worked at CDC, so I asked him what he meant. He referred me to the national salmonella database. The strain made up less than 1% of the approximately 4,000 cases in the national database. Globally, it had been found seven times from three countries in Central Africa and India, but all of these were isolated after 2000. I suspected that barely an iota of worldwide TF cases that occur annually make it into the database. The absence of a link to Carmen's homeland didn't rule out the strain's connection to the outbreak.

At the time of the outbreak, there were only two other reports of the same strain in the national database. The origin of one was missing and the other came from a Massachusetts patient in 1999. Digging further, we learned that the patient had traveled to Pakistan. We still didn't have a link but that didn't necessarily mean one didn't exist. The strain was infrequently found on two continents, conceivably its presence on a third had yet to come to the attention of public health authorities.

With the benefit of having all the data and the time to study it, I believe we did solve the mystery of TF connected to food from Malpolrica. Marcos, the missing employee, did deliveries and didn't handle food. We considered that he never existed, and that Carmen had sought to deflect blame as perhaps she had reason to suspect herself as the carrier. Marcos was young and male, two uncommon characteristics among typhoid carriers. Whether Carmen knew or suspected that she was a carrier we likely will never know. If she did, perhaps she began taking antibiotics after the inspector visited on October 5. This would explain the totality of negative stool culture results. Unless she took the recommended course for typhoid carriers, and even this is not 100% effective, she could relapse back to shedding *S. typhi* bacilli at some point after discontinuing the antibiotic. Her occasional handling of food at the restaurant during busy times, particularly if it was bare-handed, placed patrons at risk for TF and could explain the second cluster that occurred a year later. Alternatively, if a Malpolrica employee or a patron who was a food handler had contracted TF, he or she could start another chain of infections that might not be traced back to the restaurant. Ever vigilant, Sudha and her foodborne unit remain on the lookout for TF in NYC.

Typhoid Fever Cases in NYC, 1942–2020

YEAR	CASES	YEAR	CASES	YEAR	CASES	YEAR	CASES
1942	97	1965	31	1988	55	2011	26
1943	93	1966	23	1989	56	2012	46
1944	99	1967	21	1990	84	2013	23
1945	100	1968	17	1991	79	2014	39
1946	97	1969	16	1992	50	2015	40
1947	66	1970	25	1993	102	2016	22
1948	50	1971	27	1994	79	2017	37
1949	93	1972	29	1995	66	2018	42
1950	43	1973	29	1996	64	2019	36
1951	26	1974	34	1997	49	2020	20
1952	94	1975	31	1998	55		
1953	63	1976	34	1999	49		
1954	36	1977	29	2000	56		
1955	26	1978	47	2001	49		
1956	25	1979	39	2002	46		
1957	34	1980	42	2003	39		
1958	26	1981	48	2004	31		
1959	15	1982	37	2005	33		
1960	20	1983	47	2006	67		
1961	39	1984	26	2007	70		
1962	18	1985	34	2008	57		
1963	29	1986	11	2009	53		
1964	34	1987	29	2010	52		

What Has Eight Legs and Fries?

Debjani Das moved to NYC from Atlanta in June of 2000 to become a D✪D. Like Sudha, after completing her graduate studies at Emory University she worked at the CDC as a consultant for Ali Khan and virus hunter C.J. Peters on Hanta and Nipah virus epidemiology. She then transferred to skin cancer, but her passion was infectious diseases. When Debjani learned of a job opening in NYC she jumped at the opportunity to work at a local health department where she'd get the opportunity to work directly on outbreaks. Initially assigned to the Bioterrorism Preparedness Unit, she was instrumental in establishing the syndromic surveillance unit in the days following 9/11.

We were still a small bureau back in March 2001 and everyone did everything, so Debjani volunteered to take on a foodborne investigation as Sudha had her hands full with salmonella, vibrio, and the like. The call she was asked to investigate, as it often did, came from a community physician who had treated several patients who had attended the annual dinner of The Explorers Club. The club is an exclusive private club established in 1904 and is, "dedicated to the advancement of field research, scientific exploration, and resource conservation."[11] Membership is around 3,500 and was limited to men until 1981. Honorary members include Sir Edmund Hillary and Tenzing Norgay, the first persons to scale Mount Everest, aviator Amelia Earhart, and deep-sea diver Sylvia Earle.[12] Several US astronauts were purported to be members. The six-story club is headquartered on a quiet Upper East Side street in Manhattan. Website photos reveal high arched ceilings and ornately paneled wood walls that give the feel of a Gilded Age mansion. There are floor-to-ceiling windows with stained glass panels, an ivory fireplace with Greek-inspired carved figures, and another fireplace framed by two immense elephant tusks. Taxidermy on display includes a snarling hyena, lion, penguin, walrus, polar bear, and the heads of assorted members of the Bovidae family (antelope). There's even a display of rocks presumably from the summit of Mt. Everest. The club hosts an annual dinner for members and guests. This dinner was held at the Waldorf Astoria hotel in Manhattan on March 24, 2001.

The physician who called described the patient symptoms as oral paresthesias: numbing, burning, and tingling of the mouth, lips, and tongue. Others had nausea, vomiting, and stomach aches. Symptoms began shortly after the food was served with some having taken ill the following day. Debjani got a hold of the menu. The main course included a choice of sea bass, trout, or beef. There are several known toxins associated with seafood that could cause these symptoms among them ciguatera and scombroid. Ciguatera poisoning can cause oral paresthesias, vomiting, abdominal pain, and diarrhea among more serious symptoms such as bradycardia, heart block, and hypotension. Within a few hours of ingesting contaminated fish, the scombroid toxin causes a burning sensation in the mouth with flushing of the face along with systemic vomiting, diarrhea, abdominal pain, sweating, and heart palpitations. Either seemed plausible.

In ciguatera poisoning, algae produce chemical toxins and are eaten by herbivorous fish who are then consumed by carnivorous fish. The toxin is concentrated as it moves up the food chain. Fish often contaminated with the toxin include barracuda, moray eel, grouper, and sea bass. The toxin does not affect the fish, nor does it affect the fish's taste. Cooking and smoking do not destroy the toxin.

Scombroid poisoning happens in certain fish when they are stored improperly, allowing bacteria to break down tissue and create elevated levels of histamine. Histamine, as you may know, is a chemical our bodies produce during allergic reactions so symptoms like itchy skin and flushing mimic that response. Commonly affected fish include tuna, mackerel, and mahi mahi.

Sea bass was on the menu, but Debjani had a clue from the reporting physician. Many banquet attendees reported that their symptoms began right after eating appetizers and before eating the main course. Debjani turned her attention to the appetizer list and this is where things got interesting if not a little creepy. Four appetizers were served: scorpions on blue tortilla with cilantro garlic butter; roasted, spiced crickets with sweet baby corn; mealworms on snow peas with chive crème fraîche; and tempura battered tarantulas with ponzu sauce.

Consuming insects isn't just a fad evening of entertainment for wealthy globetrotters. The Food and Agriculture Organization of the United Nations released a report in 2013 outlining the prevalence, value, and future need of insects in our diet. Currently, over 2 billion people rely on insects in their diet and not because they have no other food source.[13] Entomophagy, the practice of eating some of the 1,900 edible insect species, is both culturally and culinarily acceptable in many parts of the world. The UN report makes the case that with increasing world population, global warming, and the high cost of producing animal protein—both in dollars and environmental harm— the high-protein creepy crawlers are an almost unavoidable option.[14] If you are grossed out by the thought of eating bugs I have bad news for you: Our food is contaminated by bugs. During farming, food processing, storage, and shipment, bugs get in there. There's no way to stop it. Layla Eplett, a researcher and food writer, estimates that we consume about one to two pounds of insect parts per year.[15]

More information revealed that the restaurant staff at the Waldorf Astoria did the food preparation for the 1,200 attendees. Foodborne investigations follow a tried-and-true formula. We first obtain the lists of food items served and names and contact information for the guests. This information is used to develop a questionnaire, and we attempt to administer it to as many attendees as we can reach. This is typically done by phone but with advances in technology, less labor-intensive options are becoming more common. The answers are collected, reviewed, and entered into a database for analysis—using online questionnaires has the added advantage of no data entry. The preliminary analysis compares the attack rates or percentage of sickness among persons who ate and those who did not eat each food item. The foods with the largest difference between these two percentages are implicated, but not definitive. An example presented in the following table will help illustrate this. The largest difference in attack rates is for the macaroni salad as 90% of those who ate it became ill whereas only 10% of non-eaters took ill. You might ask if the macaroni salad was contaminated how could people who didn't eat it get sick? Faulty recall or cross-contamination are a few explanations.

Example: Attack Rates of Food Consumed at an Event

FOOD ITEM	ATE FOOD AND BECAME ILL	DID NOT EAT FOOD AND BECAME ILL
Cole slaw	70%	60%
Macaroni salad	90%	10%
Potato salad	66%	72%
Tomato and basil	44%	55%

There is a second level of analysis that can be done if the data quantity and quality will allow, but the definitive link is made when the same agent is recovered from both patients and the implicated food or foods. Often there are no leftover foods and patient stool samples are challenging to obtain in time, which renders solving foodborne outbreaks challenging. Diseases caused by toxins present additional obstacles as most toxins are short-lived and testing is not readily available.

Further data analysis wasn't possible and lab testing for toxins wasn't an option, but it turned out neither was going to be necessary. The two-page questionnaire Debjani developed asked about the four appetizers; if eaten, how many; what symptoms occurred; and how soon symptoms arose after each appetizer had been consumed. The questionnaires were emailed to the guests and eighty returned them. Fifteen reported illnesses. The differences in attack rates between those that ate and those that didn't were scorpions +33, crickets -20, mealworms +20, tarantula +47. This suggested that the tarantulas might be to blame, but there was already enough suspicion cast upon the eight-legged appetizers. Eleven guests reported that the oral paresthesias began soon after consuming the tempura tarantula.

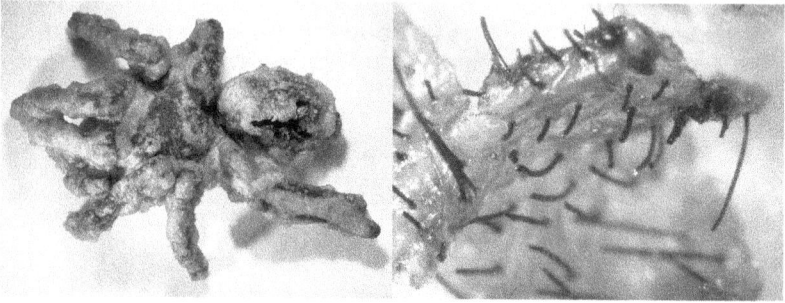

Tempura battered tarantula served at Explorers Club Dinner (left, whole tarantula, right, close-up view of setae) Photographs courtesy of Louis Sorkin, BCE, Entomologist, American Museum of Natural History

The restaurant had purchased 120 live Chilean rose-haired tarantulas from a farm in New Mexico. The female *Grammostola rosea* is about three to five inches in length while males are smaller and covered with brown to pinkish hairs. The tarantulas were stored in a refrigerator overnight to make them docile and easier to handle. The recipe called for drowning the spiders in alcohol and then carefully burning off the hairs before dipping them in batter and deep frying. The hairs on the abdomen of the Chilean rose-haired tarantulas are urticarial—cause itching—and are used as weapons in self-defense. By vibrating their back legs, tarantulas can fire dozens of their hairs at a perceived foe. The hairs, called setae, are small, less than one millimeter, with multiple barbs. A weapon perhaps the Orcs from *The Lord of the Rings* might have favored. The chemical composition of the setae is irritating to humans, and presumably also to predators. Tarantulas have thousands of setae on their abdomen and can easily be provoked to fling them like a cloud of daggers. When the setae embed into skin, they cause a local reaction characterized by redness, swelling, and itching. That's pretty mild compared to what happens if the hairs strike the eye. There's no surveillance system for tarantula-associated eye injuries, but we can get a sense from sporadic case reports. Tarantulas are often kept as pets and most injuries occur in their owners, many of whom are children. Tarantulas don't have great vision, but their bodyguard hairs are quite sensitive to vibrations and pick up sudden changes in air movement. Owners are cautioned not to breathe or blow on their tarantula as this may startle them and provoke a defensive response.

One case of tarantula setae injury that received quite a bit of publicity occurred in a twenty-nine-year-old man from Leeds, England, who visited his doctor complaining of several weeks of eye redness which had progressed to light sensitivity. An eye specialist using a slit lamp saw tiny hairs protruding from the man's cornea.[16] It was only then that the man recalled the incident. He had been focused on cleaning a stain on the glass wall of the terrarium of his pet tarantula and hadn't noticed that his pet was close by and had become agitated. By the time he turned his head, the spider had flung a barrage of hairs striking him in the face. The barbs facilitate the hairs' ability to penetrate tissues and can sometimes pass through to reach the retina at the back of the eye which can affect one's vision. Children have been injured by tarantulas kept as a classroom pet, at a birthday party, and while attending an exotic pet fair. The hairs are often too numerous and well-embedded to remove, and it can take up to eighteen months for the body's defenses to dissolve them.

An uneaten tarantula from the event was located and sent to Louis Sorkin, an entomologist at the American Museum of Natural History, for examination. He found that not all the hairs had been burned off as seen in the inserted photos. That made sense, but why were only eleven people affected? We were told that there were no other leftovers. That meant that 108 other people had presumably sampled the delicacy. A review of the cooking process found that the tarantulas were doused with cognac and placed under a broiler. A handheld blow torch was then used to singe off any remaining hairs, but some were missed. Another possibility was that others had symptoms but decided not to report them or since they lived in other countries, we didn't hear about them. Others possibly avoided the allergic reaction by not eating the abdomen where the urticarial hairs reside or were not allergic to the spider setae proteins. You might wonder about the four persons who reported symptoms of nausea, vomiting, diarrhea, and abdominal pain. It is not unreasonable to assume that they had gastronomical distress from something else eaten that night. Fortunately for The Explorers Club diners, the hairs only struck their mouths and throats, and their symptoms were short-lived. Not unlike the lives of their appetizers.

Years later, when I spoke with Debjani about the investigation, she was again living in Atlanta taking care of both a seven-month-old and her elderly mother. She recalled fondly of her days with the DꙨDs remarking that the collegiality was unmatched compared to anywhere else she had worked. "It was more like a happy family than a job."

CHAPTER 5

First Do No Hepatitis

(Dr. Westyn Branch-Elliman contributed to this chapter)

There exist within NYC, communities that feel more like a small town than a perspiring slab of metropolis. People know and speak to their neighbors, greet each other warmly on the street, and watch over each other's children. Single- and two-family brick homes with small, manicured lawns line quiet streets. There is usually one small community hospital, the kind of place where you'd likely run into someone you know, an employee, patient, or visitor. Dr. Anthony Quinlan was a board-certified gastroenterologist in just such an enclave. He specialized in endoscopy, procedures to detect ulcers and troublesome growths in the intestinal tract and remove them before they became troublesome. In January of 2000, he moved into a brand-new, state-of-the-art gastroenterology and endoscopy center in Brooklyn, the borough where he had gone to medical school and done residency training. It was home. His practice was rapidly growing as was his family. At fifty-two years old, he was a newly blessed father. Home was hectic and work demanding, but life was good.

It was in Dr. Quinlan's tranquil community, on a breezy day at the end of April 2001, that he was asked to consult on a patient at the hospital where he was on staff as a gastroenterologist. The seventy-year-old woman happened to be known to Dr. Quinlan; in fact, she had recently been to see him for an endoscopy procedure. The woman now had fatigue, vomiting, abdominal pain, dark urine, and jaundice—classic symptoms of hepatitis. She had already tested negative for the most common types of viral hepatitis—types A and B. A review of her medications and recent activities made drug or toxin-mediated hepatitis unlikely. She hadn't been tested for hepatitis C (HCV) because she didn't have any of the risk factors, such as drug use or a transfusion before blood was routinely tested. For completeness, Dr. Quinlan suggested they perform an HCV test. When the test returned positive the hospital physicians were puzzled by the results. Dr. Quinlan continued his busy medical practice but soon encountered a second, then a third patient with unexplained hepatitis. Like the first woman, both new patients were elderly, had abdominal pain, malaise, dark urine, and jaundice, and had undergone procedures in his center in the weeks before becoming ill. Neither had risk factors to explain their diagnoses of HCV. Increasingly disturbed, Dr. Quinlan could not convince himself that there wasn't a connection. He was a careful man and took his infection control training seriously. How could it have happened? He hoped there was another explanation. By the time he called the NY State Health Department to report his findings, there was a fourth case. The State referred the investigation to Dr. Layton but requested to be kept in the loop.

HCV is a virus that specifically attacks the liver. It is composed of ribonucleic acid (RNA) and is considered a blood-borne virus, transmitted by blood or body fluids, like hepatitis B and HIV. It was first recognized as a unique entity in the 1970s and was referred to as non-A, non-B hepatitis, until 1988, when it was identified as a new virus. Infection with HCV is often asymptomatic, only about a quarter of those who contract it have acute symptoms. But like hepatitis B, it can become chronic with long-term complications of liver cirrhosis and cancer. There is a lag between exposure and the onset of illness in those persons who develop acute infections. The lag, or incubation period when the virus is replicating but not causing any symptoms, is two to twelve weeks but can be as long as six months. Acute symptoms when they occur include fever, fatigue, loss of appetite, nausea, vomiting, abdominal pain, dark urine, and jaundice.

Testing for HCV at the time of the investigation occurred in two steps. First, the enzyme immunoassay (EIA) antibody test was performed to look for evidence that the body had mounted a response to the virus. The test isn't specific, meaning other illnesses might cross-react giving a false positive result. So, if positive, the test is confirmed by a more specific test called recombinant immunoblot assay (RIBA). The RIBA tests for RNA sequences specific to HCV. Persons recently infected and still incubating HCV might be negative on the EIA. A third test using PCR can be performed to detect viral RNA in such patients. However, not all HCV patients will have circulating RNA in their blood. In fact, about one-third of persons infected with HCV will clear the infection within six months. Patients positive for RNA can have their HCV genotyped, a useful method for distinguishing possible sources.

Dr. Mike Phillips had made a career and life change. Married to a surgeon and living in New Hampshire, he applied and was accepted to the CDC Epidemic Intelligence Service (EIS). EIS is a two-year public health training program for medical and epidemiology practitioners wanting to advance their skills. EIS officers are stationed either in Atlanta at the CDC or in the field at a State or City health department. Tall with blond hair and family roots in Australia, the Baltimore native had trained in infectious disease and was looking for a change of career and venue. His marriage had dissolved so when he was accepted into the EIS program he chose NYC as his assignment. Affable, hard working with attention to detail, and affectionately nicknamed Big Bird, Mike arrived in NYC in August of 2000. He was fond of saying, "You know what's interesting?" after which he would share something he had learned. He immediately fit in with the D✪Ds.

On a short-sleeved May morning, Mike and I took the R train to Southeast Brooklyn. We walked several long blocks and crossed over the Brooklyn Queens Expressway until we arrived at Dr. Quinlan's endoscopy center, a single-story building painted beige and shaded by trees. Dr. Quinlan was cordial, concerned, yet anxious. He showed us around and introduced us to the staff which numbered eleven: Dr. Quinlan, a second gastroenterologist who worked part-time, one anesthesiologist, one medical assistant, six office staff, and one housekeeping staff. At the moment of our arrival, we knew of eight patients with suspected HCV. All eight patients had an endoscopy procedure at the center during a narrow window between March 28-31. For the initial investigation, we expanded the period of interest to eight days by adding two days before and two days after the implicated procedure dates to capture any additional cases. One of our first tasks was to confirm the diagnoses and explore all explanations for the illness. We obtained appointment books, reviewed medical charts, interviewed each staff member alone, and examined the center's infection control practices.

The prevalence of HCV in New York City was estimated in 2013 to be between 1.5 and 5% in a study performed by the

D❂Ds Sharon Balter and Katherine Bornschlegel.[17] Higher rates were found in poorer communities. Worldwide the prevalence was estimated in 2016 to be 2.5%. Genotype 1 is the most common at 49% and has a worldwide distribution while genotype 3 is the second most common genotype at 18%, and is found mostly in India, Scandinavia, and parts of Southeast Asia. Genotype 4 ranks just behind at 17% and is found in Central Africa, Egypt, and Saudi Arabia. Genotype 2 accounts for 11% of cases and maps to West Africa. Genotypes 5 and 6 account for less than 5% and are found in South Africa and Vietnam, respectively.[18]

HCV is primarily transmitted by the blood of infected individuals but risk factors for contracting HCV have changed over time. The ability to screen blood for HCV in the United States began in 1992, so persons who received a transfusion prior might have been exposed, particularly in countries with high HCV prevalence rates. Persons undergoing hemodialysis are at an increased risk. Sharing needles by persons using intravenous drugs is currently the primary way the disease is transmitted. Tattooing and sexual intercourse have also been implicated. HCV is not transmissible through casual contact, not through the respiratory route, nor by food.

Nosocomial transmission, which occurs in a hospital or other medical facility, of HCV has been uncommon but perplexing when it has been documented. In the early 1990s, a cardiac surgeon in Spain who was chronically infected with HCV was found to have transmitted the infection to five patients during open-heart surgery.[19] In 1998 an anesthesiology assistant in Germany contracted HCV from a patient, and while incubating the disease, then transmitted it to five patients.[20] The anesthesiologist had a wound on his finger before becoming infected, however, neither of these episodes have been adequately explained.

We developed a set of hypotheses to explain how HCV could have been transmitted in the NYC cluster. The patients were mostly elderly, and some had immigrated to the United States. It was possible they had contracted HCV in their native countries, but it seemed unlikely. After reviewing charts and testing persons who underwent endoscopy during the last eight days of March we identified fourteen HCV positives. Finding this many previously infected, chronic HCV cases would be extremely unusual in NYC, even in a gastroenterology practice. Besides, the patients had symptoms of acute HCV. By interview, we were quickly able to rule out other possibilities, such as hemodialysis, intravenous drug use, transfusion, tattoos, and sexual transmission. That only left nosocomial transmission at the center. Had the medication vials used during anesthesia been contaminated somewhere during manufacture? The State and CDC shared that they weren't aware of any. This left five possibilities: (1) contaminated endoscopes; (2) contaminated biopsy equipment; (3) transmission during the administration of intravenous anesthesia; (4) narcotic drug diversion; (5) an unexplained breach in infection control practices as had happened in Spain and Germany.

Of the fourteen positive patients, we were able to determine through interview and medical records review that two had chronic HCV infection. One had genotype 1b and the other 2c. Of the remaining twelve patients, six were able to be genotyped, five could not genotyped, and one person refused to test. All six had genotype 2c. Sequencing of the NS5b region of the HCV genome—a molecular epidemiology technique for HCV—of five of these patients matched to the chronic genotype 2c case. We then made an epidemic curve by the date and time of the procedure. That told a more detailed story.

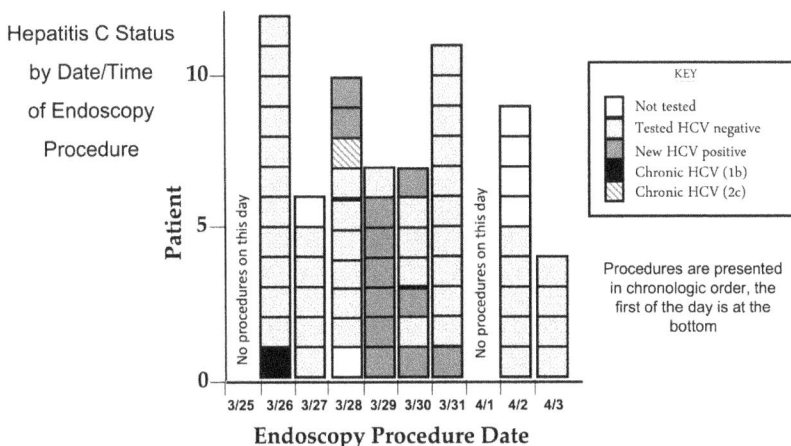

Hepatitis C Outbreak Curve by Date of Procedure chart. Created by Don Weiss

On March 26, the first patient of the day was the HCV chronic genotype 1b patient. None of the twenty-two patients who had procedures after, and agreed to be tested, were positive for HCV. Then in the late afternoon of March 28, the patient with genotype 2b HCV underwent endoscopy. The next consecutive eight patients all contracted HCV, as well as four of the eight that followed. After the first procedure on the morning of March 31 transmission ended.

If you've never seen an endoscope, imagine a black garden hose, with a smaller diameter, crossed with a Swiss Army knife. Instead of a single lumen, there are several. One for blowing air, another for water, and a third for camera and illumination. Inside the tip are retractable arms able to take tissue biopsies. One end of the endoscope is inserted into the patient and the other has an eyepiece and a connection to the power source and video recording system. Endoscopes are used for visualizing the gastrointestinal tract and there are two main types: the esophagogastroduodeno-scope, which is used to view the esophagus, stomach, and upper small intestine; and the colonoscope, which is used to view the rectum and large intestine. The center had three of each.

At our next visit to the center, we drew blood from staff to check their HCV status and observed a mock endoscopy procedure. The purpose of testing staff for HCV was two-fold. First, to identify a potential source of the cluster due to poor infection control during procedures and second, to investigate narcotic diversion. Healthcare workers are not immune to narcotic addiction. Reports exist in the medical literature of medical staff diverting narcotics meant for patients for their own use. When a person infected with HCV diverts narcotics, they may reuse the same needle and syringe used to inject themselves and introduce HCV into the remaining contents of the narcotic vial. Fentanyl, a narcotic and one of the drugs used at the center for section, is a frequently abused drug.

One staff person tested positive for HCV. She did not perform any patient care, denied drug use, and was found to have genotype 2b—not the same strain causing the outbreak. Three medications were used to sedate patients. Midazolam is in the family of benzodiazepines, like Valium, and is a short-acting sedative that has anti-anxiety and amnestic properties. The vials used contained 10 ml of the drug, enough for approximately four patients. Propofol was a relatively new drug at the time and quickly became a favorite of anesthesiologists because it induced unconsciousness but without the typical side effects of nausea and vomiting upon awakening. Vials containing 20 ml were used, enough for approximately two patients. The third drug used was fentanyl, a synthetic opioid 100 times more potent than morphine in relieving pain. The center had been using 2-ml vials, enough to treat one or two patients. In January 2001, the 2-ml vials were unavailable and were replaced with 50-ml vials, enough to treat approximately thirty-five patients.

Dr. Quinlan hired Dr. K as the center's anesthesiologist. Dr. K attended medical school in the Caribbean and was board-certified in anesthesiology. It was up to Dr. K to order and maintain all drugs and equipment necessary to provide sedation for patients. During our first visit to the center we noted that the narcotics were not stored in a locked cabinet, nor was a log of medication use kept, which are both recommended. During the mock procedure, Dr. K didn't put on gloves. He described that he would insert an angiocatheter into the patient's vein and then cap the end with an injection port. An angiocatheter is a ubiquitous device used to administer drugs, fluids, and blood products to patients. It is a long, straight, solid-bore metal needle stylet surrounded by a plastic tube, essentially a straw. The entire unit is inserted into the skin above a vein. Once the vein is punctured, the stylet is withdrawn, and the straw is inserted just a bit farther. Once the stylet is removed, blood will flow back into the catheter, and eventually out the open end if not connected to IV tubing or capped. Dr. K used infection ports, which are plastic devices that screw into the end of the angiocatheter and have a rubber port that can be accessed by needles. Dr. K reported that he did not use any extension tubing, such as a saline lock, or IV tubing with running fluids. Dr. K reported that he'd give all of the midazolam and fentanyl but would titrate the propofol to maintain patient unconsciousness. He stated that he might reenter the propofol vial for more medication, but not the midazolam or fentanyl vials.

**INTRAVENOUS
CATHETER**

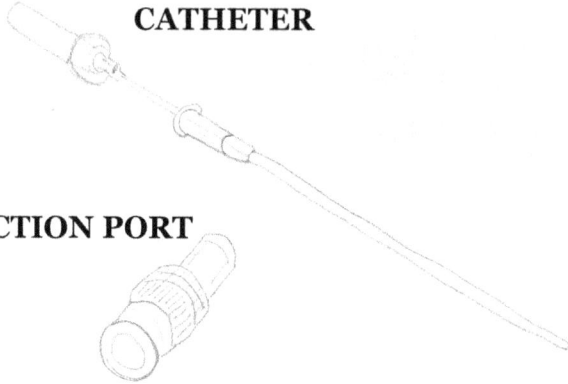

**INJECTION PORT
CAP**

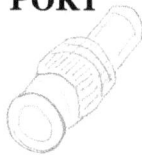

BY BROOKE BADALAMENTE

It's worth pausing here to describe medication vials and clarify terminology. A medication vial is a small glass bottle that can vary in volume from one to several hundred milliliters. The top of the vial is sealed by a metal cap that contains a rubber diaphragm. When new, the diaphragm is covered by metal and is opened similarly to a soda can. The medication is then removed by inserting a needle through the diaphragm. Single-dose medication vials are intended to be accessed once, for a single patient, and don't typically contain preservatives or anti-bacterial agents. Multi-dose vials may contain preservatives or anti-bacterial agents. These too are intended to be used for a single patient but the rule does not strictly prohibit use for several patients, as long as precautions are followed. The size of the vial alone does not indicate which type of vial it is so care must be taken to read the label, note the expiration date, access in a clean area away from patient treatment areas, and follow standard infection control precautions.

While Mike interviewed staff about their routine practices, I went with the medical assistant (MA) to witness the procedure used to re-process the endoscopes. The endoscopes were stored hanging from pegs in an armoire-like closet. The endoscopes were used in rotation and the next one for use was taken to the endoscopy suite. Nothing was done to the endoscope prior to use. After the procedure the scope is given to the MA who takes it to the sink in the endoscopy suite and aspirates tap water, then Klenzyme through the ports. The MA stated that she wears gloves throughout the entire cleaning procedure. The endoscope is then taken to the cleaning room, placed in a sink, and the exterior is cleaned with hand soap and a brush, under a stream of warm tap water.

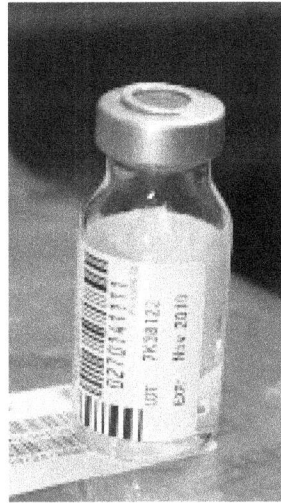

Example of a multi-dose medication vial. The vial is sealed by a metal cap which contains a rubber diaphragm for needle entry. Photo by Don Weiss

All three channels are also cleaned with a brush and tap water. Following this, the endoscope is transferred to the automated reprocessing machine, which looks like a top-loading dishwasher without the racks. Tubes are connected to the ports and the cycle takes forty-five minutes to complete. The brushes are soaked in a solution of 2.4% glutaraldehyde diluted with tap water—the amount of added water was not measured; therefore, the concentration was unknown—until the next endoscope is cleaned.

Brushes used on the outside of the scope are replaced approximately every three months and those used to clean the channels every three weeks. The glutaraldehyde solution is changed daily. Once the reprocessing cycle is complete, the endoscope is connected to a hose which blows air through the channels. A terminal aspiration of the three channels is performed with isopropyl alcohol and the endoscope is then re-hung in the closet.

After use, the biopsy forceps are wiped with a dry gauze pad, immersed in a formalin solution while in the endoscopy suite, and transported to the cleaning room where they are cleaned with hand soap and water, then immersed in the glutaraldehyde solution for approximately twenty minutes. Forceps are not autoclaved as there is no autoclave on the premises.

Mike had an idea. Since Dr. K was responsible for purchasing all the supplies, he needed to provide patient anesthesia and paid for them out of the salary Dr. Quinlan paid him, Mike reasoned that there was an incentive for Dr. K to cut costs on purchasing catheters, needles, and syringes. Dr. K used a single medical equipment supplier who was able to provide Mike with catheter and needle order invoices for the period September 2000-April 2001. During this period the center performed 1,530 endoscopies. Typically for an uncomplicated procedure, one angiocatheter, three syringes, and three needles are used. An extra angiocatheter would be needed if it clotted; additional needles and or syringes if more anesthesia was needed. During the six-month period, Dr. K had ordered 1,550 angiocatheters which aligned with the number of procedures. But Dr. K had ordered 500 needles. The minimum number of needles for 1,530 procedures was 4,590.

Mike took this line of reasoning one step further. Angiocatheter, needle, and syringe medical waste must be disposed of in a very prescriptive manner, using red sharps containers. He learned that the sharps containers were provided to the center free of charge and the MA was responsible for medical waste disposal. No records were kept regarding either the quantity or frequency of sharps waste disposal, but the MA recalled that the endoscopy suite used three two-gallons, one was still in use, two one-gallons, and one quart-size container since the center opened in January 2000. A two-gallon sharps container can hold approximately 300-400 needles plus 150-250 syringes 1-ml in size. If an angiocatheter and a 5-ml syringe take up as much space as a 1-ml syringe—which is a conservative estimate—and Dr. K had used three needles, three 5-ml syringes, and one angiocatheter per patient it should have filled approximately eighteen two-gallon sharps containers.

We invited Dr. K to our downtown office for a private interview. We picked a windowless conference room that was just large enough to fit Dr. K, his wife, Mike, and me. Mike began with softball questions—a review of the medication he used and vial sizes. Dr. K responded with the following: Propofol, 20 ml; midazolam, 10 ml; fentanyl, initially 2 ml, but then that size went out of stock, so he switched to 50-ml vials. Dr. K shared that he typically kept a two-week supply of medications in reserve. Mike then asked when the smaller vial of fentanyl again became available, why he didn't switch back. Dr. K hesitated, "I guess I just got used to them or didn't get around to changing."

Mike moved on to the issue of needles and syringes. Dr. K adamantly said he never reused needles. He repeated what he told us during the mock procedure, that he would use a separate needle and syringe for each of the three medications used. The only time he ever reinserted the needle into a medication vial after it had been in the patient was with propofol. How did he explain the lack of needle purchases? Dr. K explained that he maintained a supply of needles and syringes at his home. His wife nodded in agreement. Whenever he ran low, he would often restock his tackle box from his home supply rather than place an order. He told us he had no role in sharps disposal containers, so would not speculate as to why so few were used.

The cost of a single 50-ml vial of fentanyl is \$21.77 while one 2-ml vial costs \$2.54. If each patient requires 2 ml, then buying the larger vial costs \$0.87 per patient compared to \$2.54 for the smaller vial.[21] Recently the FDA revised its labeling criteria and both sizes are now labeled as single doses. According to the FDA, the use of the term single-dose container does not imply the entire contents of the container constitute a single dose. FDA does specify, however, that these vials are not intended for more than one patient.[22]

Returning to our list of hypotheses as to how the endoscopy patients became infected with HCV, we were able to rule out a contaminated medication from the manufacturer since no other cases had occurred at other facilities using the same lots. While the concentration of disinfectant used to disinfect the endoscopes wasn't accurately monitored, consecutive patients did not have procedures with the same endoscope. The same was true with biopsy instruments, eliminating these two hypotheses. Neither of the gastroenterologists had HCV so direct transmission from either of them could not have occurred. We found no evidence that anyone working at the center was diverting drugs and testing of the staff revealed one person, but of a different genotype from the outbreak. Neither did we find any evidence to suggest that patients had used intravenous drugs or had another risk factor for HCV, such as a blood transfusion prior to 1992, or high-risk sex, before undergoing endoscopy. None of the patients had undergone hemodialysis.

We had ruled out all the possibilities except for one: on-site contamination of multi-dose vials. A study published in 1990 explored this risk through simulation. They found that if a needle is discarded, but not the syringe, the virus can be transferred from a simulated patient to a multi-dose vial. Twenty-four percent of the doctors they surveyed used this technique.[23] Because HCV is often asymptomatic when first infected, researchers in Australia set out to see if they could identify the source for patients classified as unknown. Fifty-three of the fifty-four studied had at least one medical or dental procedure. While 20% of participants reported having sex with someone who used intravenous drugs or was positive for HCV, the researchers concluded that exposure to a medical or surgery procedure could explain how many contracted HCV.[24] An Italian gynecological surgery center had identified a cluster of HCV in 1998—four women who had surgery on the same day subsequently contracted HCV. Preceding their surgeries was a patient with known HCV, genotype 1b. All surgical personnel tested negative as did the women's sex partners. All the women had genotype 1b and the investigation concluded that poor infection control practices and use of multi-dose vial of propofol was the likely source.[25]

The fentanyl vial, being the largest, was the only vial that with a single contamination, could be responsible for the end of March cluster. Dr. K admitted he'd reenter the propofol vial but denied the same for fentanyl. It seems likely from the invoices and sharps container use that Dr. K sought to conserve needle and syringe use. Might he have drawn up the medications in the same syringe and administered them to patients? What order were the drugs drawn up and administered? Might he have injected the midazolam and or versed first, then with the same needle and syringe that had been bathed with HCV blood, entered the fentanyl vial?

The investigation didn't end there. Due to the large cluster, we expanded the investigation to look back at all procedures since the center opened in January 2000. This was a major endeavor as there were over 2,100 patients. We sent certified letters, made phone calls, and if we received no response, we sought to verify addresses and then sent another certified letter. Area physicians were notified about the outbreak and asked to help locate and test patients. However, because of the lag time from HCV exposure to the development of antibodies, patients with recent procedures were advised to get a second blood test to make sure a positive wasn't missed. Mike even made house calls to draw blood. With the help of our sister Bureau of Sexually Transmitted Diseases, we launched a site where patients could go to get free blood tests. We also expanded testing to include hepatitis B (HBV) and HIV. For non-responders, we consulted colleagues in Vital Records to inquire if the person had died. Sixty percent of the patients followed our advice and got tested, most by their primary physician.

Most of the D❂Ds were enlisted to help with the expanded investigation. They tracked certified letters and responded to those that were returned undelivered. They made phone calls and spoke with anxious patients, as well as mystified physicians. They also retrieved medical records and laboratory results. Additional help came from a student volunteer. Westyn Branch-Elliman had just completed her junior year at the University of California Berkeley. She was an NYC resident, and her mother was a hepatitis researcher at a local hospital. Westyn joined the investigation in late May and kept a diary of her experience as an apprentice D❂D. Mike assigned her to help contact patients and encourage them to get tested. Although she had experience interviewing people as a reporter for her college newspaper, she was more than a little anxious. Her effervescent personality didn't exactly lend itself to sharing potentially bad news. She dove in, nonetheless.

Patients who had received and read the certified letter mostly had already consulted with their primary care physicians and either were tested or had an appointment scheduled. Westyn arranged to get their results. The more difficult calls were to people who had not received the letter. Westyn was the first to tell them. The responses as you can imagine were quite varied. Some were frightened, and Westyn did her best to calm and reassure them.

Others were understandably angry, and they took out their anger at her, the messenger. Some suspected she was a prank caller or a lawyer from the endoscopy center. The experience deeply affected her. Westyn wrote in her diary:

> *When I started investigating the outbreak, I was thrilled. When I was in high school, I worked in a hepatitis C molecular biology laboratory and wrote a senior thesis about a sequence analysis of hepatitis C virus. From a public health stance, this outbreak is the first of its kind and possibly the most interesting public health issue to hit New York City in a decade. And yet despite my deep-seated interest in the outbreak, after a day of calling the affected individuals, I felt terrible. Unlike molecular biology— viruses and bacteria certainly don't have feelings and can't talk to you—this outbreak had a very human side. The people I called were scared, angry, confused, deceived. My feelings that the outbreak would be an interesting study in epidemiology changed quickly. Quite apart from bugs on a microscope, people are at the heart of this outbreak.*

Westyn's experience served as a reminder. Not just about sensitivity and empathy in our role as public servants, but that people, no matter how young, have important contributions to make. Remembering this has helped me connect with patients as a pediatrician as well as with adults. Sometimes all you can, and need to do, is listen.

The expanded investigation found twenty-one additional HCV-positive patients belonging to eight putative clusters. The first cluster occurred in March 2000 and the last was early in March 2001. Cluster sizes ranged from two to four patients. Sixteen suspected HBV clusters were also identified. One person tested positive for HIV but was believed to have been infected prior to undergoing endoscopy. The investigation, delayed by the events of September 11, 2001, and the anthrax letter attacks, was concluded in June 2002. The final tally was nineteen HCV cases associated with procedures at the center. There may have been more as not every patient was tested. HCV transmission was linked to the misuse of medication vials and highlights the importance of needle safety and infection control practices. The outbreak ranks as one of the most extensive and complicated investigations performed by the D❂Ds.

Mike Phillips left the D❂Ds a few years after the outbreak. He's been the chief epidemiologist for NYU Langone Health System ever since. Westyn Branch-Elliman went on to attend medical school, specialize in infectious diseases, and receive a master's degree in medical science education from Harvard University. She currently practices in the Veterans Administration hospital system.

Forty-one personal injury lawsuits were filed against the physicians and settled out of court for undisclosed settlement amounts.[26] Dr. Quinlan closed the center, and he was never accused of wrongdoing. He still practices in Brooklyn, coincidentally for NYU Langone Health System. No charges or disciplinary action was ever brought against Dr. K by the state of New York. A review of the NYS Department of Education website reveals that he is not licensed to practice medicine in the state. At last check, he no longer practices anesthesiology but does practice medicine in a neighboring state.

CHAPTER 6

Death by Post

Spore Noir

The call came in late afternoon on October 29, 2001, from a Manhattan hospital. A possible 10-24, that's an assault. The victim was a sixty-one-year-old woman. She was in the ICU and in bad shape. From what the doctors said it was likely to become a 244, that's murder with an illegal weapon. I didn't bother to ask what illegal weapon, instead my partner, D✪D Nash, and I headed straight up there. The silver-haired doctor led us through the ICU to an isolation room window. On the other side was a woman hooked up to a maze of tubes and wires. She was badly swollen but without any evidence of wounds. There was a tube connected to a ventilator breathing for her and she was heavily sedated. We weren't going to be able to interview her, not unless she recovered.

"Who is she?" I asked.

"Kathy Nguyen. She works as a stockroom clerk at Manhattan Eye, Ear, & Throat Hospital (MEETH)."

The doctor led us to a lightbox and slid in a radiograph. Nash was new on the force and he looked puzzled. It was a chest radiograph. The heart and cardiac structures appeared white in the center left. Typically they occupy two-fifths of the diameter of the chest cavity. In the image we were staring at, the whiteness was more than half the diameter, crowding out the blackness of the air-filled lungs. The lungs didn't look so good either, blotched with white from either displaced fluid or blood.

"Widened mediastinum," I told Nash.

We followed the doctor down to the lab where he directed us to a microscope. Nash looked first. He gasped. I adjusted the focus and took a look. A tangled mess of blue thread met my eyes. I'd stared down the barrels of microscopes quite a bit in my years before joining the department but had never seen anything quite like it before. The doctor dripped a drop of oil on the slide, then flipped to high power, adjusted the focus, and motioned us to look again. With the increased magnification the thread no longer looked continuous, instead, it was made up of segments. Embedded within the segments were clear zones where the stain had not been taken.

"Spores," I said.

I asked the doctor where he got the sample.

"Blood," he replied.

"When?"

"Last night, when she came into the emergency department, about 11 p.m."

I checked my watch, it was almost six. It had taken less than eighteen hours for the bacteria to grow—another clue.

"We need those samples," I said. The doctor obliged and ran off to package them for us.

Nash turned to me, "Another late night."

I grunted and nodded. Neither of us voiced what we were thinking—that this changed everything. The pace of the past seven weeks was about to kick into another gear. We headed back downtown, first to drop off the samples at the lab, and then to the office with the medical records to brief AC Layton and to begin to sort out this latest threat.

After the Al Qaeda attack that destroyed the World Trade Center and killed 2,996 people, we were on high alert for a follow-up attack. Bioterrorism was our concern, and we created an early warning system in hospital emergency departments to detect illness from a covert biologic release. The theory promulgated a few years earlier was that any single clinician might not recognize an illness due to a biological agent because the early symptoms resemble mundane illnesses, like the flu. If, however, a large number of patients—that number wasn't known then and still isn't known—came to different emergency departments across the city with the same or similar complaints this "signal" could be detected and a response initiated. The goal of the system, called emergency department syndromic surveillance, was to detect early cases that were unusual in their timing, volume, or geographic location. With this information, we could administer antibiotic prophylaxis or vaccine, depending on the agent, to the exposed and prevent serious consequences. In the weeks after 9/11, we chased many syndromic surveillance signals, but none panned out to be a concern.

But some person, or perhaps persons, had done the unimaginable. Like the plot of a Cold War spy novel, a deadly bioweapon had been unleashed. It was anthrax spores. Some of the recovered spores were so pure they floated on air. We thought only a state-sponsored bioweapons program could have grown and refined anthrax spores to be used in this manner. But as the cases accumulated throughout October 2001, it seemed less likely international, and more likely domestic. The targets were peculiar too. A tabloid newspaper in Florida, network news anchors, and NYC newspapers. The route, too, while unanticipated, was not surprising. Ordinary number ten envelopes via the US Postal Service. We eventually learned that a limitation of the syndromic surveillance was that it was designed to identify serious illnesses, like inhalation anthrax. We didn't anticipate that the first cases of bioterrorism would be the cutaneous form of anthrax.

Television and print news offices receive hundreds of letters each day. Some are tossed, others are opened first before they are discarded, and some letters are saved for a stock reply. In late September 2001, staff who handled incoming mail at the *New York Post*, NBC, and CBS noted skin infections on their hands, face, and chest walls. They sought medical attention and were treated for the usual causes. A baby brought to her mother's office at ABC during a birthday celebration developed a sore on the upper arm the day following the visit. Once anthrax was discovered in a Florida photo editor the NYC patients had their infections re-evaluated. All, plus three others from the *New York Post* and NBC, were diagnosed with cutaneous anthrax. Several recalled opening suspicious letters with granular powders.

The first letter recovered was found at NBC and was sent to Tom Brokaw. It was addressed using all capital and block lettering and bore no return address. The postmark date was 9/18/2001 and was mailed from Princeton, NJ. The powder was described as a mix of brown sugar and sand. It was assumed that similar letters had been mailed to Dan Rather at CBS, Peter Jennings at ABC, and the editor at the *New York Post*. Of the three, only the letter to the *New York Post* would be found.

By mid-October 2001, the CDC knew of ten anthrax cases, and only the two in Florida were the more serious inhalation type. One person had died. The five NYC cutaneous anthrax cases all had gotten sick on or before October 1, so it seemed that the attack might be over. One contaminated letter had been found and another was suspected to have been thrown away. Mailrooms were taking precautions, yet two more cases would be found in

New York Post workers who had searched for a letter. The city was still gripped with white powder mania, seeing anthrax at the bottom of cereal boxes and in the residue inside gum wrappers. Maybe soon we'd be able to breathe easy again.

In the afternoon of October 22, the other spore dropped. It was announced that four postal workers in the District of Columbia and New Jersey were ill with inhalation anthrax. Two had died. That's when the focus of the investigation shifted from persons receiving anthrax-tainted envelopes to anyone in the delivery path of mail. DOD Nash was sent to the lab to help them deal with the influx of white powder samples. I was assigned to accompany two CDC epidemiologists en route to the NYC post office facilities.

The US Postal Service is a massive operation. Most people don't give a second thought to how it operates and manages to deliver over 400 million pieces of mail each day in congested cities and rural outposts. The workhorses of the system are cancellation and sorting machines. Incoming mail, such as a first-class letter, is first processed through cancellation machines which cancel the postage, add a postmark, add a location black bar code to the front, and an orange tracking bar code to the back. The black code is more specific than a zip code and helps direct the letter to your local postal carrier. On bulk mail, you can see it under the address in the window. The orange bar code is used to record the time and location of the letter through every machine in the system. You probably never noticed these barcodes and you might miss the orange one if you don't look closely.

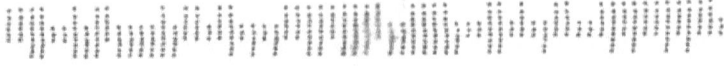

Delivery Bar Code on the Front of an Envelope.

Rear Tracking Bar Code.

Another series of machines, called the delivery bar code sorters (DBCS), read the front code and sequentially sort the envelope, first to the correct postal office, and then into a bin that is specific to your mail carrier. The machines reminded me of the IBM punch card sorters I worked with in high school. I'd grab a stack of rectangular cards filled with punch holes and load them into a tray. Based on the instructions keyed in, the cards would get sorted according to the pattern of holes. To keep the machine running smoothly the cards, and in the postal world, envelopes, have to be neatly stacked and held tight by a spring-loaded device. Letters passing through DBCS are subjected to squeezing forces as they pass through the rollers and guides. Compressed air hoses extending from the ceiling are used to clear dust from the machines. Large fans blow in an attempt to keep the area cool. Why bother to explain all this? The machines and codes will become important later in the story.

Kathy Nguyen died on October 31, 2001. *Bacillus anthracis* was confirmed in her blood. There didn't seem to be a motive for anyone to want to kill her. No enemies. No jilted lovers. She didn't gamble or owe anyone money. She didn't trust banks and paid all her bills by money order. She'd cash her paycheck, then go to a check cashing outlet or the nearest post office to get the money orders. Ms. Nguyen wasn't involved in any nefarious activities. Whatever exposed her to anthrax spores appeared to be random, but how and where was she exposed? Where she lived? Worked? Were there spores out there waiting to infect others? Was she collateral damage or was the intended victim of a test release? The investigation was no longer just ours. A team of NYPD, FBI, CDC, EPA, USPS, and departmental staff began dissecting her life and daily routine.

Kathy Nguyen was born in Vietnam and immigrated to the United States in 1977. Her life was typical of many New Yorkers. She went to work, attended church, and enjoyed shopping, food, and friends. She was soft-spoken but engaging and was liked by her coworkers and Bronx neighbors. Ms. Nguyen bought food and gifts for friends. She lived in a third-floor rear apartment not far from the 6 train in a residential Southeast Bronx neighborhood that was predominately Latinx. She was not wealthy and had no immediate relatives in NYC. Reportedly a son had died in a car accident and an ex-husband lived across the country in California. There might be a sister in Texas. Many described her as a loner.

Data from Ms. Nguyen's Metro card was retrieved and told us the dates and times she entered the subway, but not when and where she got off. Regardless, this allowed us to piece together much of her movements in the days before she became ill. She worked the evening shift at MEETH, arriving often early for her 2:00 p.m. start time. Her job was to receive supplies, maintain the stock room, and distribute equipment throughout the hospital. The stockroom was in the basement, adjacent to the mailroom.

Ms. Nguyen spent some of her free time at a Macy's store in Parkchester, in Chinatown, and in stores and restaurants in the Upper East Side of Manhattan where MEETH is located.

Interviews with coworkers turned up a clue: Ms. Nguyen's sought medical care on October 25 because of eye irritation. She hadn't recalled or mentioned a specific incident and attributed it to the usual dust in her workspace. A nurse irrigated her eyes and thought nothing more of the episode. We sought to learn what Kathy Nguyen had in common with the other cases.

Robert Stevens worked as a photo editor at a tabloid newspaper run by American Media (AMI) in Boca Raton, Florida. He was the first case of anthrax diagnosed in the outbreak. When it was announced on October 4 that he had inhalation anthrax it was quickly dispelled by federal officials as a fluke and due to a natural exposure. Mr. Stevens was an outdoorsman, he fished and hiked. Anthrax spores can be found in soil and often find their way onto animal hides. Later it came out that Robert had handled several suspicious envelopes containing unknown substances. That was the beginning of distrust in the information the government was providing. Soon after it was announced that anthrax spores were found on his computer keyboard, in the building's mailroom, and that coworkers had tested positive. A person from the AMI mailroom also had inhalation anthrax.

MEETH was closed when I arrived on October 29. It was close to 9 p.m. and security was holding back a crowd of television crews and wasn't allowing anyone to exit. NYPD and our staff were gathered outside the building. Dr. Joel Ackelsberg was trying to negotiate an agreement so we could proceed with the investigation, but the police wanted assurance from us that the place was safe for their personnel to enter. We couldn't give them that assurance. The standoff lasted several minutes until D✪D Sharon Balter announced that she was going in, and "If we find anthrax, I'll just take cipro." We all followed. Department staff quickly organized a point-of-distribution clinic to hand out ciprofloxacin.

I interviewed a close friend of Ms. Nguyen's who shared that she spoke little English, traveled to Chinatown once a week, and had made a trip to visit Ground Zero on October 7.

By midnight the makeshift clinic was in full operation. We set up on the second-floor mezzanine and used portable curtains to interview staff semi-privately. An assembly line system was employed to hand out ciprofloxacin tablets. The interview form was long, and the line moved slowly. My job was to circulate and answer medical questions, but the trouble was we didn't have any answers. People wanted to know their risk. We didn't know how or where the exposure occurred. Was it even in the building? And how many spores did a person have to inhale to get sick? Was it the same for everyone? Or were some people more susceptible? And for how long did the spores remain suspended in the air? Once settled, could the spores re-aerosolize?

I'd been in a similar predicament two and a half weeks earlier. On October 12, a letter with white powder was opened at *The New York Times* office by reporter Judith Miller. Her desk was in an open bullpen-style room with a dozen or so other desks. The powder had gotten on her desk, skirt, and a favorite sweater. The police wouldn't let anyone leave the building since it was a potential crime scene, but this only multiplied the already high level of anxiety. I was escorted by a NYPD detective into the lobby packed with *Times* staff. The crowd wound up the staircase to the second-floor landing. My task was to speak reassuring words. The worst thing a public health official can do is give people false information out of ignorance. That destroys not only your own but the entire department's credibility. Best to be honest and confess to that which you don't know. All I could do was assure them we'd be sampling and getting them the information as quickly as possible. We didn't know how well spores could be distributed by opening an envelope. At that point, none of the contaminated letters had yet been recovered. All we had to go on was what had been reported from Florida. Just one person, the one who presumably opened the spore-laden envelope, in a similar office space, got sick, or so we thought. And there were antibiotics to prevent infection if exposed. Perhaps I was a bit too reassuring, but fortunately, the letter was a hoax and did not contain anthrax spores.

I'm not sure the staff at MEETH were reassured. They had access to antibiotics, though a sixty-day course of ciprofloxacin was not without its risks. Environmental sampling was conducted with a focus on the stock and mail rooms. The stock room was small, perhaps twelve by twelve, and filled with shelving. Some supplies were stored in the boxes they were shipped in. Nothing suspicious or out of the ordinary was found upon inspection. Many swab and wipe specimens from both locations were rushed to the lab. All were negative for anthrax.

Investigators in HAZMAT suits searched Ms. Nguyen's apartment. They took her mail to test and swabbed her mailbox. No spores were found. All the building tenants were interviewed. One tenant reported a nasty sore on her thumb that wasn't healing. Testing involved taking a biopsy and sending the specimen to the CDC lab for examination. That too was negative. Both Ms. Nguyen's home and work neighborhoods were canvassed door-to-door. We had a photo of Ms. Nguyen's to show each proprietor and worker asking each if they recognized her and when they last saw her. We went to area churches too. We didn't learn anything more than we already knew.

What little we knew about how weaponized anthrax might behave came from an incident that occurred in the Soviet city of Sverdlovsk, now Yekaterinburg, in 1979. Sverdlovsk is about

1,500 km east of Moscow in the Ural Mountains and while dot-
ted with farms the town was the location of a clandestine Soviet
bioweapons plant that manufactured powdered anthrax. In late
March, a plant supervisor removed a filter for cleaning—but did
not replace it. The filter prevented spores from drifting out of the
plant's exhaust stacks into the air. The next shift failed to notice
the missing filter and started up the next production run. At first,
the Soviets said there was a natural source outbreak in livestock
and that humans got sick from eating and handling contaminated
meat. They claimed there were no inhalation cases. After the
dissolution of the Soviet Union, the truth emerged—sixty-four
people had died—most from inhalation anthrax, and a map of
cases followed the prevailing winds, tracing a neat, aerosol plume
that stretched four kilometers. The final case count may never
be truly known, but likely exceeded 100. Four kilometers is over
two miles. For the spores to have traveled that far they had to
be aerodynamic and couldn't have been clumped. Animal studies
suggested that the LD_{50}, the dose at which 50% of people die, was
somewhere between 2,500 and 55,000 spores. The downwind victims in Sverdlovsk couldn't have inhaled many spores, suggesting
that the minimum infective dose might be much lower.[27]

Marci Layton and I joined an environmental team making a
return trip to Kathy Nguyen's apartment on November 11. For
the first visit on November 1, investigators donned hooded, Tyvek
suits, gloves, booties, and face-covering respirators. Nary a spore
was found so we entered this time in street clothes. Other than
bags of clothing and shoe boxes, the place was neat if not sparse.
Next to a twin bed covered by a floral-print blanket was a small
beach chair and foldable table, the kind one might use to eat dinner in front of a television. Two of the windows were guarded
by heavy metal gates as they led to the fire escape. On the sill of

the third window was a cactus plant. There was a small desk and lamp. Most of her mail had already been taken, but we found an unopened letter from the MTA. Among a dozen or so business cards in the desk drawer was her social security card. There was also a photo of a young groom in a white tuxedo. Holding onto his left shoulder was his smiling bride wearing a flowing white gown, the bottom of which spread the width of the photo. They posed next to a vase of flowers. Another photo was of an older woman, in a blue shirt riding in a wooden cart with a thatched roof building in the background. There were several twenty-dollar bills and lottery tickets. Toothpicks still in their plastic sheaths. There was a pad on which it looked like someone had started to write a letter with a date printed at the bottom: 7.28.1990. The refrigerator was stocked as if waiting for its occupant to return to cook dinner. These were the fragments of a life meaninglessly cut short. More swab and wipe samples were collected.

Again, no spores were found at Ms. Nguyen's apartment. The local post office that processed mail for Ms. Nguyen's building was also tested for spores. It too was negative. The outbreak had grown to twenty-one cases—eleven were the cutaneous type and ten were inhalation. Four people had died, two were postal workers. Several weeks had passed since Ms. Nguyen's illness with no new anthrax cases or leads in the investigation. Spores, however, continued to be found around the globe. At US embassies that had received mail or diplomatic pouches from Washington, DC; Lima, Peru; Vilnius, Lithuania; and Yekaterinburg, Russia. Spores were found in eleven offices in the Hart Senate building and two in the Russell Senate Building. Mailrooms at the Supreme Court, Walter Reed Medical Center, the Department of Veteran Affairs, and Howard University were positive. A videotape sent to the mayor of NYC from NBC was viewed suspiciously and it too tested positive. Multiple samples from NJ, DC, Maryland, and Virginia post offices, including four DBCS machines at the NYC Morgan facility, tested positive.

There was yet another level of uneasiness simmering below the surface that government officials were forced to face once they learned that no spores were found either at the hospital where Kathy Nguyen worked or at her home. It was a long-standing fear that threatened not only the welfare of New Yorkers but also their livelihoods and the city's economic welfare—the subways. Shortly after 9/11, we implemented a system to monitor MTA workers as a way to detect a public release of a biological agent. We found no absences that were suspicious for anthrax. This, along with the absence of any new cases in several weeks, reassured city leaders that the testing was likely to turn up nothing but would serve as a reassurance for riders that the system was safe. The carefully crafted plan tested five stations used by Ms. Nguyen and four stations that she neither used nor intersected with the lines she did use. Health Commissioner Neal Cohen happily announced on November 17 that the tests were negative.

Unfortunately, the outbreak wasn't over yet. In a small, Central Connecticut town, in a modest house on a quiet street, lived Ottilie Lundgren, a ninety-four-year-old widow. She no longer worked or drove and left her home infrequently to visit the library, hair salon, and church. Friends and relatives took care of her needs and accompanied her on physician visits and to a local diner. She read often and watched television. She received assistance to pay her bills, which she opened by slitting the top with a letter opener; bulk mail solicitations were torn in half and tossed into the trash. On November 13, 2001 she became ill with flu-like symptoms. It worsened and three days later she asked to be taken to the local hospital. Similar to Kathy Nguyen, she progressively got worse and developed respiratory distress. She died from anthrax on November 21. Connecticut's health department investigated, obtaining hundreds of swabs, wipes, and air samples from her home and all the places she had visited. Like with Ms. Nguyen's case, none tested positive for anthrax.

Suppose one morning I wake up and purchase a powdered sugar donut from the corner bakery and eat it on the way to the subway. I'm a messy eater and get powdered sugar on my hands, coat sleeve, and pants. I then get on the subway and brush up against other commuters along my way, each of whom has a different route and destination. When I grab the overhead bar, I transfer some powdered sugar. When I sit, more sugar is left on the seat. Suppose each contact transfers powdered sugar to another commuter. Some of the people I contact, or who've contacted items I've touched, in turn, brush against other commuters further spreading the powdered sugar. The powder enters offices, schools, and hospitals. Some commuters are heading to towns in New Jersey or Connecticut, they contact others on those transit lines as well. While other commuters go to the airport to fly to another city or even another country. They spread the powder to people they contact on the way to the airport and the planes. People getting off those planes spread the powder along the routes they travel. All of us would continue to spread the powder until there was no smidge of sugar left to spread. This is what we were dealing with but with anthrax.

Letters moving through the postal system move analogously as commuters through mass transit. In the hypothetical example above there would be no way to track where the powdered sugar from my donut ended up. The US Postal Service employs an electronic system that tags and tracks mail. When first-class mail passes through the cancellation machine, the back of the envelope is stamped with an orange bar code. The code then is scanned and recorded so that the path and time of the letter as it moves through the system are known. Bulk mail is treated differently but can also be tracked. However, the data isn't saved forever. The postal distribution centers in Florida and New York where anthrax letters passed through had not saved the data from the dates in question. But the Brentwood (DC) and Trenton (NJ) facilities had. No letter from either facility was directly delivered to either Kathy Nguyen's or Ottilie Lundgren's home. The USPS tracked 300 letters that were processed at the same time as the letters sent to Senators Daschle and Leahy and were delivered to the Bronx. Unfortunately, none could be recovered to test for anthrax spores.

However, two letters were identified that passed through the same Trenton sorting machine three hours after the Daschle and Leahy letters and arrived at the Wallingford processing center in Southern Connecticut. Neither had been delivered to Ms. Lundgren's postal route nor were recovered for testing. Another letter passed through the Trenton sorting machine 283 letters after the Leahy letter was delivered to an address four miles away from Ottilie Lundgren's home. The letter was found and the outside, but not the inside, tested positive for anthrax. Testing at the Wallingford USPS facility found four DBCS machines were positive for anthrax. One machine, #10, which was used to sort bulk mail, was heavily contaminated. Machine #6, used for a final sort, had a positive result in the bin specific for Ottilie Lundgren's postal route.

The similarities in the cases of Kathy Nguyen and Ottilie Lundgren prompted us to compare notes. Both women lived alone and led quiet lives with predictable daily routines. Testing in their homes turned up no spores. There was one more thing that the two women shared in common. They both owned the same brand of perfume. One of the theories we entertained was that a terrorist might fill an atomizer with anthrax spores and anonymously spray people as they pass on busy NYC streets. As any New Yorker can tell you, city streets are filled with the unusual. Aside from panhandlers, you'll encounter sidewalk vendors with tables full of burning incense, hats, and used books; people reciting Bible verses, others speaking loudly with no visible cell phone, men and women wearing sandwich boards upon which they've scribbled manifestos, among others. The perfume bottles tested negative for anthrax.

The mail cross-contamination theory of exposure, although the theory of last resort, was not without supportive evidence. Spores from the letter opened in Senator Leahy's office were disseminated throughout the Hart building. When 642 garbage bags of quarantined mail addressed to the Capitol were examined in a specially sealed warehouse, sixty-two bags were found to have a trace amount of spores, five bags yielded 100 cfu/liter of air, and one bag had over 750 cfu/liter of air. That bag had the unopened letter addressed to Senator Daschle; the only letter found in the bags.[28]

A Canadian study released weeks before the anthrax mailings used nontoxic *Bacillus globigii* spores to simulate what would happen in a typical mailroom. They placed 0.1 grams of spores on an 8.5 x 11 sheet of printer paper and folded it into thirds. The paper was placed in an envelope and sealed only with the envelope's adhesive. The letter was shaken and mixed in with other identical, but empty letters so that the opener would not know which one contained the spores. When the letter was opened in an eighteen-by-ten-by-ten-foot room with typical ventilation, the spores quickly disseminated to all corners of the room and remained detectable in the air for the full ten minutes of observation.[29]

The fate of Georgi Markov was also on our minds. Markov was a Bulgarian ex-patriot, dissident, writer, and critic of the Soviet Union working for the BBC. He lived in London and in 1978 while waiting for a bus, he felt a sharp pain in the back of his leg. He turned to see a man carrying an umbrella walking away. Four days later, Georgi was dead. The umbrella-gun-assassination device, built by the Russians, delivered a platinum-iridium pellet filled with a lethal dose of the toxin ricin. Was the Russian-made umbrella gun just one weapon in their bioweapons cache? Was anthrax in NYC a test run of yet another weapon?

There was scant evidence linking a person to the mailed letters as there were no fingerprints on the envelopes. The FBI was able to test all the mail drop boxes that would result in a Princeton postmark and one on Nassau Street, across from the Princeton University campus, tested positive. But there were no eyewitnesses who saw the person that mailed the anthrax-tainted letters. Nor was there a confession. The FBI was under tremendous pressure to solve the case and prevent subsequent acts. In desperation perhaps the FBI submitted a sample from the Leahy letter for carbon-14 dating. The results placed the spore creation date sometime between 1998-2001 and came with many caveats. The information did little to advance the investigation.

The CDC then employed suspect profiling to identify the anthrax mailer. Who had access to the anthrax and a motive? Dr. Steven Hatfill worked at the US Army Medical Research Institute of Infectious Diseases (USAMRIID), the lab where bioweapons were studied, in the late 1990s. He had lived and attended medical school in Rhodesia, now Zimbabwe, where he studied anthrax outbreaks. Dr. Hatfill was alleged to have boasted that he knew how to weaponize anthrax and developed training materials for soldiers to recognize mobile bioterrorism labs, in anticipation of the invasion of Iraq.[30] Several people in the bio-weapons community thought him a credible suspect and told the FBI as much. The FBI initially replied that he had an alibi but was eventually convinced to take another look at Dr. Hatfill. The suspicions were fueled because he reportedly had the skills and possible motive to be the anthrax mailer.[31] He had recently filled several prescriptions for ciprofloxacin, the recommended drug to prevent anthrax if exposed.[32] From a pond near his home in Maryland was retrieved a device that was thought to be a portable glove box capable of being used to fill letters with spores, but was shown to have no connection to the investigation. Dr. Hatfill also knew how to scuba dive and the FBI postulated he filled the letters underwater to prevent his own exposure. Another clue that allegedly implicated Hatfill was that there's a community called Greendale in Rhodesia. Greendale was the name of the fictitious school written on the return address of the anthrax-laden letters sent to Senators Daschle and Leahy. The evidence against Hatfill was circumstantial at best yet led the FBI in the wrong direction.

Dr. Hatfill's apartment was searched several times and each time the media was alerted, and a circus atmosphere ensued. On one occasion a specially trained bloodhound ran up to Dr. Hatfill, causing handlers to assume the dog smelled anthrax on him when it was more likely bacon from breakfast. The FBI searched his father's and girlfriend's homes. They even employed aggressive "bumper-lock" surveillance, in which the FBI followed him so closely to give the impression that their bumpers were locked together. The FBI also directly accused (ultimately incorrectly) him of murder. As a result, Dr. Hatfill was fired from his job and lost his security clearance. The FBI then tapped his phone and got him fired from another job before he even started. Local police got in on it, pulling him over for alleged minor driving violations.

Attorney General John Ashcroft called him a person of interest on national television. The FBI was certain they had found their man, and the media was relentless. Many of Dr. Hatfill's friends and colleagues abandoned him, and the few who didn't, worried that he'd take his own life to escape the torment.

Many of us in the public health and medical community knew it was going to take science to crack the case. The last two decades have seen exponential advancement in DNA sequencing technology. The Human Genome Project was completed in 2003 as a result, a bacterial genome can be sequenced and assembled in a matter of hours. This allows rapid comparisons of human and environmental specimens during disease outbreaks similar to comparing a fingerprint from a crime scene to a database of known offenders. On October 4, 2001, the FBI, with the assistance of Dr. Paul Keim, an anthrax expert at Northern Arizona University, identified the anthrax used in the Florida mailing as the Ames strain. The Ames strain is believed to have originated from a deceased cow in Texas. The exact provenance of the specimen is debated but was likely sent to the National Veterinary Services Laboratory in Ames, Iowa, which sent it to the USAMRIID where it was identified as a new strain and given the name Ames.

The identification of the Florida anthrax as the Ames strain was done by sequencing a fraction of the approximate 5.5 million base pair genome of *Bacillus anthracis* and comparing it to what at the time was a very limited database of anthrax genomes. Knowing the strain was Ames was analogous to a witness being able to say the suspect was a White male, five foot nine to eleven with brown hair, and driving a car with California license plates. It narrowed down the sources, but not nearly enough. But there was something else they noted when working with the spores from the letters. Bacteria placed on artificial media grow as colonies. If skillfully plated, each round dot is one colony, and the character-istics, such as color, size, and texture, are specific to the bacteria. When the spores were grown in culture some colonies looked different. This suggested that these differences might be genetic in origin—mutations that could be used to definitively identify their origin.

There were perhaps dozens of labs in the United States, and likely more throughout the world, that possessed the Ames strain. Al Qaeda couldn't be ruled out, nor could the Russians. In fact, it would be clever for a foreign terrorist group to use an American-origin anthrax strain to cast suspicion away from themselves. The FBI produced a list of fifteen US labs and three foreign labs that held Ames strains. How they came by this list and its comprehensiveness was a question. They subpoenaed the labs requesting samples of all their Ames strains. The work began in May 2002 and involved the FBI and four contractor labs. They first compared the letter strain to the original Ames strain and identified four mutations in the letter strain that were not present in the original Ames strain. The second phase began in May of 2002 and took five years to complete. The scientists had to create probes for the four mutations. A probe is a sequence of DNA that is the mirror image of the sequence of interest. Using the technique of PCR, the probe is added to a solution containing the DNA of the unknown strain. If the sequence is present in the sample, then the probe anneals (attaches and the sequence is multiplied until it reaches a level that can be detected. It took time to validate the probes and then test the 1,070 Ames strains that had been collected. Only one strain, found in several labs, had those four mutations. Its origin was a flask labeled RMR-1029 in a USAMRIID lab.

The creator and owner of that flask was Dr. Bruce Ivins who

had been advising the FBI as an anthrax expert during the investigation. The focus then shifted away from Dr. Hatfill and onto Dr. Ivins. The evidence against Bruce Ivins was circumstantial. He worked late into the evenings at the lab in the weeks before each letter mailing, and as it was later revealed, this was his habit throughout his time at USAMRIID. The FBI wrote in their final report that his motive was fear of losing his life's work. The anthrax vaccines he was developing had not performed well and he feared that funding would end. The FBI reasoned that Ivins believed an anthrax attack would force Congress to continue to fund his research. To some colleagues, Dr. Ivins was an odd duck, with curious mannerisms and obsessions. And he had mental health issues. One of his obsessions was the Kappa Kappa Gamma sorority and there was an office near where the letters were mailed in Princeton, NJ. But colleagues doubted he could have produced the weapons-grade spores, and certainly not in one week, which is what the FBI asserted. The main evidence against him was his ownership of the murder weapon—flask RMT-1029—and that he allegedly misled investigators when they requested Ames samples by sending a false sample supposedly from the flask. The sample tested negative for the four mutations.

In a *FRONTLINE* exposé that aired in 2011, a fellow researcher at USAMRIID shared that he had submitted several samples of RMR-1029 from his lab that tested negative for the mutations. The FBI disputes this. The National Academy of Sciences (NAS) was asked to convene an expert committee to review the science the FBI used to identify RMR-1029 as the murder weapon. Their report, published in 2011, casts doubt on the FBI's certainty.[33] Four of the suspected seven anthrax letters had been found but not all of them were checked for the mutant variants, as the FBI claimed. They believe the suggestion that Ivins deliberately sent a false sample was overstated. Ivins and a coworker, prepared samples together and sent them to both the FBI and Paul Keim. The FBI rejected and discarded the sample because Ivins used homegrown media and not commercial media as instructed. Ivins resubmitted the sample. The original sample stored in Keim's lab tested positive for all four mutations, the repeat sample did not. If Ivins had something to hide, why would he send the correct first sample and decoy the second time?

Furthermore, when the RMR-1027 flask was subjected to an experiment where it was sampled thirty times, only sixteen times did all four mutations test positive. The sensitivity of the assays to detect the mutations was also called into question. The NAS expert committee also took issue with the FBI anthrax repository and the testing performed. All samples were voluntary, so if a lab had something to hide there was no check of compliance. Labs frequently share materials and record keeping wasn't always complete. And what about foreign labs of countries that are not US allies? Only labs from three countries, Canada, the United Kingdom, and Sweden, submitted strains to the FBI. The Ames strain has been in use in laboratories since 1981. Is it possible that Russia, China, North Korea, and Iran didn't get their hands on it? Of the 1,070 strains that were collected by the FBI, only 957 yielded usable results for the mutations. That's like a criminal investigation not bothering to consider 113 suspects just because they didn't answer their phones.

Among the evidence the FBI turned over to NAS for review were reports of a suspected Al Qaeda bioweapons lab in a foreign country. On three occasions the US government sent teams to the site to get samples and from all three they detected anthrax DNA, once finding the Ames strain. The FBI took it further, testing the remains of a hijacker from Flight 93 for anthrax. One assay was positive, but the FBI discounted the result as laboratory contamination.

In March 2024, a Russian memo appeared in news stories describing a "non-lethal sonic weapon." Some experts believe this is the source of Havana Syndrome, the brain injuries suffered by US State Department employees and their family members. Considering the FBI's zeal and pursuit of Steven Hatfill based on flimsy circumstantial evidence, from which he was later proven innocent, and the Russian proclivity to use weapons to achieve political goals, can we be sure that Bruce Ivins was the anthrax killer or a convenient fall guy?

Did Bruce Ivins have the technical skill and equipment to produce spores of the refinement used in the anthrax letters? After all, no spores were ever found in his home or lab. We learned in 2006, when a natural case of inhalation anthrax occurred in a man using animal skins to make African drums in NYC, that spores spread easily and are difficult to eliminate. Were the anthrax-laden letters sent by a foreign terrorist group or government? We likely will never know for sure. Bruce Ivins died by suicide in 2008 and Steven Hatfill was exonerated. The federal government reached a settlement in Hatfill's defamation lawsuit for $5.82 million. It seems likely that Kathy Nguyen and Ottilie Lundgren both contracted anthrax from a minimal number of spores that had arrived on cross-contaminated mail.

CHAPTER 7

Pain From a Pain Clinic

Unless you have the rare genetic disorder of pain insensitivity you've experienced pain. And likely often. Who hasn't had a headache, stubbed toe, or sunburn? Those pains are fortunately short-lived. However, chronic pain, lasting three months or longer, is often a debilitating condition. The Institute of Medicine estimated that 116 million US adults, about two in five, experience chronic pain.[34] Pain is big business, not just for the pharmaceutical industry, but for clinicians. The projected global revenue from treating chronic pain in 2024 was more than $100 billion.[35]

The human body is equipped with specialized sensors called nociceptors whose function is to convert noxious stimuli, be they physical, chemical, cold, or heat, into an electrical signal. Nociceptors are distributed throughout the body. The electrical signals are relayed through the spinal cord to the brain where they are converted to the sensation we perceive as pain. Pain is an early warning system designed to identify harm and cause an action to avoid the stimulus and prevent tissue damage. If you put your hand in a flame, the heat triggers a nociceptor signal to the brain to move your hand.

Pain is sometimes called the fifth vital sign. But unlike blood pressure, pulse, respiratory rate, and temperature, there's no way to measure pain, short of the imperfect question, "On a scale of one to ten, how much does it hurt?" While we all feel pain, we don't experience it quite the same. Pain threshold is defined as the length of time it takes a person to perceive a stimulus as painful while pain tolerance is a measure of how long the pain can be endured before an action is needed.

Joint pain caused by osteoarthritis (OA) affects over 30 million Americans. The joints most often affected are the ones that bear the greatest gravitational forces, namely the knees, hips, and spine. Cartilage wears away and bone rubs against bone causing unrelenting pain and the limitation of activity. In the spine, the cushions between the vertebrae can be forced out of position and impinge on the nerves exiting the spinal column that innervate the legs. Sciatica, a vexing pain that radiates down the back of the leg, can result.

Pain has always been part of the human experience, and our ancestors were aware of natural substances that possessed analgesic properties. The latex of the poppy plant, *Papaver somniferum,* was known to the Sumerians of Mesopotamia over 5,000 years ago to induce euphoria and sleep.[36] Willow bark, which contains salicylate, the chemical basis of aspirin, was used to treat pain and fever. Pre-Columbian inhabitants of Peru chewed coca leaves to relieve pain and fatigue.[37] In the sixteenth century, Paracelsus dissolved powdered opium into wine and named it laudanum, an analgesic that enjoyed widespread use for centuries, despite its addictive tendency.[38] Aspirin has been around since 1897, acetaminophen has been available commercially since 1950, and ibuprofen since 1969. Newer opiates came on the market in the 1980s and 1990s, most notably oxycontin, which has resulted in an epidemic of abuse and overdoses. What all these drugs share is that they can be taken orally, however, when taken orally, they first need to be absorbed, then distributed via the bloodstream to the location of the pain.

When the drug enters the bloodstream, it doesn't just go to the location of the pain but is distributed throughout the body. This results in side effects and can potentially damage non-target organs. Meanwhile, the body seeks to eliminate the drug, either through direct excretion or metabolizing it into an inactive form. To treat localized pain, for example from a back injury, you must take a large enough dose of the drug to get enough to the location of the pain to have an effect. And once the drug reaches the intended target, there's nothing that keeps the drug there or from being broken down.

The use of injections to treat localized pain evolved with the invention of the hollow-bore needle and syringe in the 1840s and 1850s. During the early part of the twentieth century, regional nerve blocks were discovered, and the first joint injection may have employed cocaine. It wasn't until the 1950s that intra-articular injections with corticosteroids became popular. While medicine hasn't found a way to prevent OA, and there's no cure short of joint replacement, the availability of pain control treatments has mushroomed in the last several decades. Pain treatment centers, medical facilities operated by trained clinicians administering evidence-based therapies, should not be confused with opioid pill-mill dispensaries. The latter swaps pain for addiction, exploiting patients for profit.

Infection following joint injections is reportedly a rare complication, as long as well-established infection control measures are followed. These include handwashing; wearing of cap, gown, face mask, and gloves; disinfection of skin, and sterile techniques. Face masks weren't a routine recommendation until clusters of

Streptococcus salivarius, a bacterium that lives in the human mouth, caused cases of meningitis in women who received spinal anesthesia during childbirth.[39] The anesthesiologists who performed the procedures are believed to have contaminated the needles or sterile field with oral secretions. Similarly, caps are needed to prevent contamination from falling hair or skin cells.

As often happens, this cluster of infections was brought to the attention of the department by a community clinician. The infectious disease physician taught medical residents at two Brooklyn hospitals and noticed that each facility had admitted a patient with bacteremia—bacteria in the blood. She called Dr. Layton at 5:00 p.m. on Friday, October 17, 2008, and shared that both patients had the bacterium *Klebsiella pneumoniae* in their blood and underwent pain-relief procedures at the same outpatient pain treatment center (PTC) on the same day. Had the doctor only known of one patient, she might have not been concerned enough to make the call.

The following Monday, October 20, we began the investigation by calling the PTC and speaking with Dr. T, the owner and sole practitioner. He was cooperative and revealed that five recent patients had contacted him to report either increased pain or fever following procedures performed on October 13 and 14. Dr. T instructed all five to be evaluated in the nearest emergency department. I asked Dr. T for an overview of the procedures and medications used. He described a typical injection for sciatica whereby the patient lies on their abdomen on a table and the overlying skin is then disinfected with betadine. Lidocaine is then injected to numb the skin at the site of the injection. Dr. T used a small amount of radiopaque dye under fluoroscopy, live image radiography that appears on a screen, to localize structures and position a 22-gauge spinal needle into the desired location.

Attached to the needle is an extension tube connected to a syringe filled with a steroid medication to reduce swelling and control inflammation and an anesthetic for immediate pain relief. The steroid used was triamcinolone and the anesthetic was bupivacaine. I inquired with Dr. T about the medication vials—how many doses each contained and whether they were being used for multiple patients. He explained that the triamcinolone was prescribed for each patient and came from the New England Compounding Center in 10-ml vials. What about the bupivacaine and radiopaque dye? Here it got more complicated. He had bottles of different sizes and couldn't recall which were used when. We'd have to sort this out in his office by examining his records and supplies.

Dr. T was instructed to cease using multi-dose vials and preserve any open vials of medication or dye for the department to collect for analysis. He was further instructed to fax to the department the names and contact information of all patients treated on October 13 and 14, contact all the patients who had reported symptoms to check on their status, and notify the department of any other patients with post-procedure complications. We scheduled the site visit for the next day. With the help of Public Health Nurse Paula Del Rosso, we began the tedious task of collecting information on patients. I spoke with the physician who had reported the two cases to Dr. Layton and Paula retrieved medical records. The first patient was a sixty-two-year-old man who underwent injection of the sacroiliac joint on October 13, 2008. He received injections of dye (3.5 ml), followed by a mixture of bupivacaine and triamcinolone (total volume 4.0 ml) into the left sacroiliac joint at 2:15 p.m. Forty hours later he had chills, a temperature of 102°F, and pain that made it difficult to walk. He was admitted to a local hospital where a culture from his blood grew

Klebsiella pneumonia. He was treated with antibiotics for five days and recovered.

The second patient was a thirty-six-year-old woman who also had a sacroiliac injection for back pain resulting from a car accident. She received the same two injections of dye and a mixture of bupivacaine and triamcinolone (total volume 4.0 ml) into the left sacroiliac joint at 4:00 p.m. on October 13. The next morning, she had a headache and pain at the injection site, followed soon after by fever, chills, and malaise. In the emergency department, her temperature was 104.4°F and she rated her pain at ten on a scale of ten. A blood culture likewise grew *Klebsiella pneumonia.* She remained hospitalized on antibiotics for one week and recovered.

Among the three new patients were an eighty-one-year-old woman with *K. pneumoniae* bacteremia, a forty-three-year-old woman with *K. pneumonia* in her urine, and a seventy-one-year-old woman who had similar symptoms but no bacteria in her blood or urine. All three had sacroiliac injections on October 14.

One case of bacteremia immediately following a pain injection could be explained by a mishap. Such as poor skin preparation or a patient with risk factors for infection. Three blood-borne infections, and we did not yet know if there were more, suggested a systemic problem. Among the infection control mistakes that sprung to mind were needle or tubing reuse, poor hand or sterile prep hygiene, and contaminated multi-dose vials. Multi-dose vials have been an ongoing concern and linked to several outbreaks, both in NYC and throughout the world. While they might be economical, the repeated need to puncture the diaphragm risks the introduction of foreign material, such as bacteria and viruses.

Back in 2002, a pain clinic in Oklahoma made the news when seventy-one people contracted hepatitis C (HCV) and thirty-one got hepatitis B (HBV) following treatment. Investigators determined that a staff person had administered intravenous anesthesia to patients and reused the needles and syringes.[40] The needles and syringes had become contaminated by the blood of chronically infected HCV- and HBV-infected patients when inserted into intravenous tubing. Three years later, in the fall of 2005 in Massachusetts, seven people contracted *Serratia marcescens*, a bacterial infection, after receiving injections for pain. This time investigators, which included future D⊗D Alison Ridpath, determined that a multi-dose vial of contrast had been contaminated.[41] Over the years 1983-2002, twenty-seven outbreaks linked to multi-dose vials occurred and were reported in the medical literature.[42]

We checked with the CDC to learn of any other recent occurrences of bacteremia following pain injection procedures in the United States. They hadn't but suggested that we check if a compounding pharmacy was used. Compounding pharmacies are middlemen that take drugs from manufacturers and mix them into formulations, doses, or packages most convenient for clinician use. The New England Compounding Center had prepared the triamcinolone medication used. When I called, they denied any problems with product contamination but agreed to examine the medication lot provided to Dr. T.

Melissa Wong was a Council of State and Territorial Epidemiologists foodborne fellow. She joined the investigation and developed the chart abstraction tool and patient interview form. The first aim was to identify other PTC patients with post-procedure complications, direct them to seek emergency medical care if they hadn't already, and examine if any particular procedure was associated with bacteremia. These data points would help identify the infection control error, or errors, requiring correction.

Melissa and I were accompanied to PTC by Lisa Heine and Ronnie Volpe, department nurses with expertise in infection control. We arrived at 2 p.m. and were ushered into Dr. T's office as he was in the middle of a procedure. He poked his head in and invited us to observe the procedure, a radiofrequency ablation (RFA), which uses radio waves that produce heat to interrupt nerves sending pain signals to the brain. Dr. T wore gloves and a lead apron, but no mask, cap, or sterile gown. A man lay face down, undraped, on the procedure table. His jeans were positioned an inch down his hips. The characteristic brown of betadine was not visible on his skin. It could have been wiped off, but typically this isn't done until after the procedure, and often there are telltale stains that remain. Protruding from the right side of the man's lumbar spine were four 22-gauge needles. None of the needle ends were capped or had the stylus in place. Sequentially, Dr. T. inserted the RFA probe into a needle, adjusted the voltage, administered the dose, and then after removing the probe injected a mixture of bupivacaine and triamcinolone. His assistant held the medication bottles for him should he need to refill the syringe.

We had hoped to review the medical records of patients seen on the days in question, but Dr. T had not yet completed his procedure notes. As the hour was late, we'd have to make a return visit to review records and conduct a full infection control inspection. We confiscated the lone opened 10-ml vial of triamcinolone (4 ml), along with five unopened triamcinolone vials, and opened vials of bupivacaine (30 ml), and iodixanol (100 ml). After completing the chain of custody forms, the medications were delivered to PHL, where they began the process of determining whether bacterial contamination was present.

We returned to the PTC on October 23 to conduct the full, infection control practices investigation. We were fortunate that

Lisa and Ronnie were able to make the return visit, as the more eyes, the better. Site visits are the public health equivalent of a crime scene investigation. But instead of looking for blood stains and splatter, we look for adherence to blood and body fluid precautions. Instead of shell casings, we look for medication vials, how needles are discarded, and how syringes are used. Our investigation searched for DNA, but bacterial, not human DNA. We retrieved from the hospitals the bacteria and their DNA from patients' blood infections. The smoking gun would be finding matching DNA somewhere among the instruments or medications in the office. But what to sample? On the floor of the treatment room was a nearly full, red sharps container. I peered in and saw an assortment of spinal and ordinary injection needles. Retrieving needles was too dangerous and likely low yield as I doubted the lab had a protocol to test needles. We could collect surface swabs, but from where? We already had the medication vials, so the only additional samples we collected came from the hand sanitizers. In France, in 2006, there was an outbreak of *Serratia marcescens* in a neonatal intensive care unit that was tracked to a contaminated liquid soap dispenser.[43]

Infection control investigations are detail-oriented and tedious. A three-dimensional, Where Did Waldo cut corners, get sloppy, or ignore rules? The office was shared with a gastroenterologist and Dr. T's space consisted of five rooms: a waiting area, two consultation/exam rooms, one of which doubled as Dr. T's office, the preparation and recovery room, and the procedure room. One consolation room was leased to a cosmetologist who performed hair electrolysis. Medical records were stored in cabinets in a hallway. We did a room-by-room inspection, with five sets of eyes looking into every nook and corner. Lisa and Melissa had a checklist that we all followed. We opened cabinets and moved equipment to peer behind. We looked in the refrigerators and opened drawers, all the while jotting down notes and nodding to each other. Each staff person was interviewed separately. We verified the licenses of Dr. T and his MA.

We also had Dr. T perform a mock procedure, analogous to recreating a crime. Dr. T was instructed to do exactly what he would do if this were an actual procedure. He entered the procedure room and donned a lead apron, a precaution since the fluoroscopy machine emits radiation. Dr. T didn't wash his hands with either soap and water or hand sanitizer. The lead apron was visibly soiled, and he couldn't say when it had last been cleaned. The mock patient's skin was cleaned with betadine followed by covering with a sterile drape. Dr. T didn't wear a mask, a recommendation when doing such procedures, nor a cap to keep hair from falling onto the patient. To access the joint space, Dr. T preferred that the tip of the 22-gauge spinal needle be at a 45-degree angle. The needle he used came in a commercially produced spinal tap kit and was straight. With gloved hands, Dr. T bent the tip of the needle to the desired position. To draw up the medications he had his assistant hold medication bottles upside down and with a needle and syringe, Dr. T withdrew the quantity of dye needed. He repeated with a second needle and syringe to withdraw the bupivacaine followed by the triamcinolone. A sterile extension tube was removed from its packaging and attached to the syringe and spinal needle. First, the dye would be injected, and the position of the spinal needle adjusted using fluoroscopy until it was positioned correctly. The syringe with the dye was then removed and the medication syringe affixed to the tubing. At this point the medication would be injected, the needle and drape removed, skin cleaned of betadine, and a Band-Aid placed over the injection site. The needles and syringes were ultimately disposed of in a sharps container located on the floor.

Before leaving for the day, we presented Dr. T with a list of immediate corrective actions and followed up with an official letter detailing the complete list of twenty-five corrective actions. These included handwashing before and after each procedure, before and after each patient examination, using the standard surgical scrub technique of up to the elbows; a face mask, cap, and a gown over the lead apron are to be worn when performing procedures; all medications should be single-patient-use only and no vial should be used for more than one patient and entered as fewest times as is necessary; injection sites should be thoroughly cleansed with betadine and the betadine should be allowed to dry before beginning the procedure; spinal needles should not be bent with hands or left open to the air when not being used to inject medication; the stylets should be kept sterile and replaced; the sharps container should be emptied when two-thirds full and not kept on the floor; medication names and lot number need to be recorded in the patient's charts; the procedure table and countertops should be cleansed after each patient; and lead aprons should be cleaned after each procedure but at least daily.

The PHL results came back the following week. All the unopened medication vials were negative for bacteria, as were the used vials of triamcinolone and bupivacaine. Bacteria were cultured from the bottle of iodixanol dye, and the organism identified was *Enterobacter aerogenes*. However, the three patients with bacteria in their blood had a different bacterium, *Klebsiella pneumonia*. While the lab results didn't connect a medication contamination to a sick patient, they were not surprising. Our first visit to PTC had been on October 21, seven days after the implicated procedures. The triamcinolone vials contained 10 ml. The usual dose was 1 ml per patient, so each vial was enough for ten patients. The bupivacaine bottle held 30 ml; at 2 ml per patient, it would last fifteen patients. Dr. T treated an average of six patients per day, therefore each medication vial would not last more than a few days.

The iodixanol bottle contained 100 ml and Dr. T typically used 1 ml of iodixanol per patient. The 100-ml bottle could last a month. Upon questioning, Dr. T shared that after he learned of initial patients with infections, he discarded the open vials of triamcinolone and bupivacaine on October 15 and the iodixanol vial he was using on October 17. The vials we confiscated were not the ones used on the day the patients were infected, at least we didn't think so. Regardless, the presence of bacteria in the vial of dye was indicative of an infection control lapse. The lab had retrieved the patient cultures from the hospital laboratories and had begun to compare the bacterial DNA among the three patients. The question we sought to answer was if the patients were infected by a common source.

We kept on interviewing patients and searching for additional cases. Since English was the second language for many of the patients, we made use of our Russian-speaking staff. DOD epidemiologists who assisted included Anna Smorodina, Inna Katsovich, Sara Sahl, Raj Sunkara, Fazlul Chowdhury, Cherylle Brown, José Poy, and Lucretia Jones. We didn't have to wait long to learn of additional patients. The day after we learned of the lab results, Melissa and I were back at the PTC to abstract charts. Several hours later as we exited, bleary-eyed and hungry, the office informed us that a new case connected to the PTC had been reported. The patient, a fifty-eight-year-old woman, had a sacroiliac injection on October 17. The day after the procedure she experienced pain and made several visits to the emergency department before the diagnosis was made. Her blood culture grew *Enterobacter aerogenes.* Yes, the same species PHL had isolated from the bottle of iodixanol dye. *Klebsiella* and *Enterobacter* are inhabitants of the human intestinal tract.

The new case required additional and immediate action. We could not be sure there weren't ongoing risks to patient safety and therefore could not allow Dr. T to continue to administer injections. I began drafting a Commissioner's Order which was delivered to Dr. T on October 30. The order directed Dr. T to cease injections until we had completed our investigation, and the infection control recommendations were satisfactorily implemented.

To facilitate the identification of affected patients, we drafted a health alert. The Health Alert Network (HAN) was conceived by Dr. Layton to communicate information, often urgent, to the NYC medical community. It began as a fax system to hospitals and outpatient medical centers but evolved to utilize email and a website. Any provider can sign up for the service. The HAN of October 28 was targeted at lab and hospital staff who may have encountered a patient in the preceding weeks and detailed the current situation. We asked that they search their medical and lab information systems and report to the department any patients who recently had bacteremia with either of the two organisms or a link to the PTC.

Dr. T performed several different procedures to treat musculoskeletal pain. The location of the injection depended on the perceived nerve source of the pain. We reviewed the records for fifty-nine procedures performed from October 13–28 as Dr. T was ordered on October 28 to stop procedures until all corrective actions were completed. We were able to interview fifty-four patients or their proxies. The most common procedures performed were transforaminal lumbar epidural injection, sacroiliac joint injections, greater femoral trochanter bursa injections, and medial

branch block. Nine patients had symptoms suspicious of an infection following their injection and four had proven bacteremia. The
patients had injections between October 13–24 and all nine had
sacroiliac injections.

Our colleagues in the PHL, Lillian Lee, John Kornblum, and
Yin Lin, had taken the samples we'd dropped off and cultivated
bacteria from one vial. Using PFGE, they were able to match the
Enterobacter aerogenes DNA patterns from the iodixanol vial and
the patient. Furthermore, the *Klebsiella pneumoniae* DNA patterns
from the three patients with blood infections were indistinguishable. We had links proving a connection between an infected
patient and a contaminated medication vial, and that the other
three patients had a common source for their infections. It was as
close as we've ever come to a smoking gun, or vial as it were, in
infectious disease investigations.

The bags of skin sanitizer we removed from the patient intake
and procedure rooms had been sent for analysis. Nothing was
cultivated. We were able to track the volume of hand sanitizer
used and it didn't add up. Based on the volume of patients the
hand sanitizer supply should've needed replenishing, but two
were nearly full, and one was only half empty. The New England
Compounding Center submitted their report which found no
bacterial contamination of the triamcinolone lot. They would not
be so lucky a few years later when the country's largest outbreak
of fungal infections was linked to them.[44] A pharmacist was
sentenced to eight years in prison for intentionally misbranding
products and ignoring safety regulations, among other crimes.[45]

In all, we made seven visits to the PTC, the final visit was
six months after the outbreak had ended. During that visit, we
noted that multi-dose vials were still in use. Our authority over
this practice was limited as the FDA has authority over drugs. We

enlisted the assistance of then NYC Health Commissioner Tom Frieden who sent a letter to the FDA Commissioner highlighting the need for regulations on the use of multi-dose vials.

Interventional pain management is a growing field. In part, because people are surviving longer than their joints. However, a worrisome trend is the average age of people receiving knee and hip replacements is declining.[46] Obesity, physical inactivity, desk jobs, and working from home all contribute to musculoskeletal decline predisposing people to osteoarthritis. At the other extreme, sports-associated injuries and overuse also contribute to the growth of the interventional pain industry. The societal move away from chronic dependence on opiates will further have patients seeking alternative therapies.

The business of intra-articular pain injections is expected to grow by 7% over the next decade.[47] While much has been done to strengthen and alert practitioners about infection control practices, only one state, New York, requires providers to complete training as part of licensure renewal. Unfortunately, the situation with multi-dose vials hasn't changed much. In 2018, the FDA issued non-binding recommendations about medication vials. The recommendations are about labeling, not use. There is a national surveillance system to monitor healthcare-associated infections that is focused on hospitals, nursing homes, and dialysis centers. The system does not include pain treatment centers unless they also perform surgical procedures. It remains difficult to detect outbreaks connected to pain treatment centers. It behooves consumers to be cautious, shop around, ask questions, and verify infection prevention practices before choosing a pain treatment provider. A check of the New York State Office of Professional Medical Conduct website revealed that Dr. T has never been subject to disciplinary actions.

CHAPTER 8

On the Trail of a Serial Killer

Serial killers live and work among us. They are fathers, husbands, and members of our communities. Consider the Gilgo Beach suspect, Rex Heuermann, an architect and family man whose DNA has allegedly been found with a victim's remains. Heuermann has pled not guilty to the charges against him.[48] The BTK Killer, Dennis Rader, was a home alarm system installer and was caught through the testing of his daughter's pap smear DNA.[49] The motives of serial killers are often vague, and the attacks appear random, but they have a modus operandi and patterns.

The bacterium *Neisseria meningitidis*, also known as meningococcal disease or MD, behaves similarly. It lives among us, mostly in harmony, and appears to attack at random. Serial killers often have nicknames that are self-appointed or dubbed by the media or law enforcement. So, does MD. The media has dubbed it spinal meningitis, which is just one of several syndromes it causes. While the reign of serial killers ends when they age, die, or get caught, MD's rampage continues. Like in the movie, *Time After Time*, in which the story of Jack the Ripper merges with the H.G. Wells novel, *Time Machine*. MD the serial killer transcends time. In the twelve years before I joined the D❂Ds, MD attacked 615 New

Yorkers, killing 104. A case fatality rate that exceeded tuberculosis and all BCD-monitored diseases.

Fortunately, serial killers are rare, and so is MD, which occurs in about one in a million of the US population over the past decade. Yet it wasn't always the case. After World War II, with American soldiers returning and an influx of refugees, the rate of MD was closer to one per 10,000. From the beginning of the collection of disease surveillance data, MD has victimized the very young and old. Case rates have been highest in individuals under four years of age and rise again in those over sixty-five years of age.

N meningitidis is also a peculiar organism. It runs the spectrum from a deadly illness to an innocuous, unnoticed colonizer of the nose and throat, with its disease occurrence dependent on the strain and the individual. The bacterium is readily passed from person-to-person by respiratory droplets. Most people are temporary hosts. The bacterium resides in their nose or throat for a few weeks, and they eliminate it and develop immunity. The technical term is colonization and there are no symptoms, however, those colonized, as well as infected persons, can transmit the bacterium to others, particularly their household contacts. A small proportion of individuals get ill when the bacterium enters the blood which causes one or more syndromes including bacteremia or blood poisoning, sepsis, meningitis, and pneumonia. While treatable by common antibiotics, MD can trigger an exaggerated response by the immune system resulting in rapid death in 10–15% of those infected. That's a high death rate for an infectious disease in industrialized countries and why MD has a feared reputation as a serial killer.

My first encounter with the serial killer MD came in high school. Spinal meningitis terrorized families, panicked parents, and frightened kids worse than visions of monsters hiding under the bed. It was the wintertime of my freshman year in high school. The newspapers—in the 1970s this was the way people learned of local events—had created anxiety by reporting that a high school student had died from spinal meningitis. The boy had been on the wrestling team and the local board of health—this is a common misnomer, health departments do this work, not their oversight boards— was working to identify any kids who had been in contact with the child. They also pushed erroneous messages about how the disease is transmitted which resulted in wrestling mats across the county getting sanitized. MD is transmitted by respiratory droplets. It does not survive long in the environment. The aforementioned carrier state complicates control efforts. At any given moment, 5–15% of the population host *N. meningitidis* in their nose or throat. The strains vary and the percentage of carriers differs by age. Carriers can pass the bacterium to others, who themselves are unlikely to get sick. Eventually, the bacteria find a susceptible host and causes illness. It is nearly impossible to track the path back to the person who infected them. Think of the Kevin Bacon saying that any actor can be connected to him through movies in six steps, but instead of six degrees of separation, it is more likely dozens if not hundreds of degrees of separation between MD cases.

We happened to be doing wrestling in ninth-grade gym class at the time and were pairing up for matches. My opponent looked across at me. There was more than concern in his eyes. He was terrified. He wasn't athletic and I outweighed him by a few pounds, but it soon became clear that losing or pain wasn't what worried him. It was the mat. When the whistle blew, he quickly rolled over on his back so I could pin him, and he could get off the mat. A few years later another case of MD made the local paper. This time it hit closer to home. A high school basketball player from a neighboring town who I peripherally knew from pickup games at the town courts had died of MD. He was seventeen years old.

Early in the evolution of the D❂Ds, one of the organizational changes that came about as BCD grew was to assign diseases to designated subject matter experts. It was like picking players to be on your kickball team at recess, or fantasy football team. I knew my choice: *Neisseria meningitidis*. Maybe I chose it because it's rare or because of its seriousness. The public health response is urgent, which reminded me of my days working in the pediatric emergency department. Or maybe because there are control measures and a vaccine. The choice was likely also influenced by my experience in medical school and the way it moves silently through populations. I couldn't name the major reason and suspected there were other, perhaps subconscious ones. As subject matter experts, it's our responsibility to keep up with the literature, track the epidemiology trends in NYC and the world, review protocols, oversee case and outbreak investigations, advise the department, and serve as spokespersons for media inquiries.

While MD had been an enigma in high school, I was in the last month of my fourth year of medical school when I believed I had come face-to-face with the disease. I was doing an elective in pediatric infectious disease at the children's hospital in Newark, NJ. Admitted to the ward was a four-year-old girl named Ethel. She had meningitis and everyone suspected MD. I read articles and books to prepare the case report and presentation on rounds. *N. meningitidis* is a fastidious, meaning fussy about nutrient requirements, gram-negative bacteria. It doesn't hold the blue stain used to identify bacteria and will appear red under the microscope. It's a diplococcus, appearing as two bacterial cells smushed together like biscuits baked in too small of a pan. *N. meningitidis* virulence in part is due to an outer, waxy, capsule that

allows it to evade the immune system. It is classified by the capsule into twelve serogroups, denoted by letters. Most infections
are caused by six serogroups: A, B, C, W, X and Y. Ethel recovered, and it turned out she wasn't infected with *N. meningitidis*
after all, her meningitis was caused by a related and rarer bacteria
called *Moraxella catarrhalis*. I wouldn't forget what I had learned
about MD and years later, when I worked in the St. Louis City
Health Department, I lived in constant dread of an outbreak. We
had limited resources to respond to outbreaks.

The public health response to MD is to identify close contacts and offer them antibiotic prophylaxis to prevent illness and
subsequent transmission. A single dose of ciprofloxacin, an oral
antibiotic, can reduce the chances of an exposed person contracting disease by several hundredfold. The problem is that there's no
easy way to tell who is really exposed. So, we err on the side of
caution and prophylax more people than likely need it. In the last
year ciprofloxacin resistance in *N. meningitidis* has necessitated
changes in prophylaxis in NYC and other parts of the country.
Adaptability, as detailed in the following pages, is a feature of *N.
meningitidis*.

The identification of close contacts has been the responsibility
of the public health nurses (PHN) team of the D❂Ds. It is delicate work and requires superb communication skills, sensitivity,
and perseverance. Close contacts include sex and drug-sharing
partners, subjects most people prefer to keep private. If the patient
is unable to be interviewed due to the severity of the illness or
death, then the PHNs interview the next of kin. The relative may
know little of their loved one's private life so credit card charges,
cell phone logs, and online dating app profiles often prove useful in identifying persons in need of antibiotic prophylaxis. The
PHNs use a structured interview form to ask questions and record

the information. The form undergoes periodic review as diseases and risk factors evolve. The critical interview technique employed by the PHNs was to get the person comfortable enough to talk about their life. Questions not on the form often led to discussing activities that identify people at risk—weddings, funerals, as well as illicit activities. The database we were using in 2006 had fields for the basics, such as demographics, but not the questions included in the MD form. A limitation that made it difficult to detect subtle connections promptly.

The name *N. meningitidis* has caused some confusion among the public, the press, and even some doctors. *N. meningitidis* can cause meningitis, but also pneumonia and bacteremia. By far the most serious complication of MD is called meningococcemia, a form of bacterial sepsis with a high mortality rate. The commonly held belief repeated by the media is that MD causes only meningitis. This thinking has led the public and medical providers to fail to consider MD in the absence of the symptoms of meningitis. This is a mistake, often a deadly one.

Obtaining bacterial cultures from sick persons is important for case identification, serogrouping, and DNA fingerprinting of *N. meningitidis*. Prior to 2020, the DNA fingerprinting technology available to us was PFGE. Bacteria are grown in culture, and the DNA is extracted, and digested using a restriction enzyme that cuts the strand into fragments-based sequences. The fragments are placed on an agarose gel and subjected to a shifting electric field. This causes the fragments to migrate based on size and charge creating a band pattern loosely resembling a vertical bar code. Then software analyzes the pattern and compares it to previous patterns returning a percent similarity. The CDC arbitrarily defined ≥ 85% as the related strain threshold. PFGE seems crude by comparison to the WGS tools available today, however, it was useful in defining outbreak-associated cases.

A polysaccharide-based vaccine for MD serogroups A, C, Y, and W was approved in 1978, however, the indications for use were limited. Because of the rarity of the disease, only persons with certain risk factors or who were traveling to high-incidence countries were recommended to receive the first MD vaccines. There was no vaccine for serogroup B, which was the primary attacker of young children. Furthermore, while the vaccines protected adults, they were far less effective in young children. It wasn't until 2005 that new vaccines utilizing conjugate technology were approved in the United States and became part of the routine childhood vaccine schedule—first for adolescents and then added to the routine childhood recommendations.

The other important thing to know about MD is that it can cause outbreaks. In Sub-Saharan Africa, there is an area called the meningitis belt because it frequently suffers large MD outbreaks during the dry season. When I arrived at BCD there hadn't been an outbreak in NYC as far back as anyone could remember. That was about to change in November of 2005. A Bronx woman had traveled to Brooklyn to visit her boyfriend. A few days later she became ill and was diagnosed with MD. At first glance, the Bronx woman wasn't unusual. The serogroup was C, which was common; she survived, and none of the contacts she shared with us became ill. Secondary cases weren't typical. We hadn't seen a secondary case among a close contact in many years, likely the early 1990s, before my time at the department. In part because MD infected a vulnerable subset of the population and because we actively offered antibiotic prophylaxis to contacts. The investigation was unable to identify how she had come in contact with the bacterium. Her case was classified as isolated and sporadic.

During the following month, four more MD cases appeared.

MD is a somewhat seasonal disease, occurring more often in cold weather months, so this alone wasn't alarming. At the time there were thirty to forty MD cases a year in NYC: roughly five to twelve cases per quarter. In 2005, there were a total of twenty-eight cases, the lowest number since 1993. What caught our attention was that three of the four new MD cases were also serogroup C, one could not be serogrouped, and they all occurred from just a few zip codes in Brooklyn. The usual pattern in NYC was one-third each of serogroups B, C, and Y distributed throughout all five boroughs. PHNs Susan, Paula, and Kate picked up on another commonality: recreational drug use kept coming up during their interviews. To complicate matters, the hospitals, perhaps lulled into complacency by the declining number of cases, had failed to report cases in a timely manner. The first and fourth of the December cases had been roommates, so we had a secondary case. Because we hadn't been notified in time, we weren't able to offer prophylaxis. A missed opportunity to prevent a secondary case and were concerned there could be an outbreak brewing.

As previously mentioned, *N. meningitidis* is a fastidious organism. It doesn't survive long in the environment and is quite sensitive to antibiotics. Anyone suspected of having MD should be treated immediately with antibiotics without waiting to obtain diagnostic testing. These facts render the recovery of *N. meningitidis* from patient specimens difficult. The limitations in detection meant that cases often went undiagnosed and interventions such as close-contact prophylaxis went unapplied. Antigen tests of spinal fluid were available, but at least half of the MD infections didn't involve the nervous system, and not all hospital laboratories stocked the kits. Antibiotics had to be given quickly but treatment just as quickly rendered blood cultures negative.

At the risk of getting too far into the medical weeds, the *N.*

meningitidis capsule can disrupt the immune system and cause a dramatic loss of platelets and clotting factors. The development of a rash is common. The rash at first may appear as flat red areas that blanch or fade with pressure but then the rash becomes petechial, meaning that blood vessels have leaked and left pinpoint blood stains trapped in the skin. As the immune system overreacts, platelet and clotting factors decrease, and patients bleed, externally and internally. You may have seen people with large purplish bruises called ecchymosis, they often appear in elderly people who've had blood drawn. In severe MD, petechiae increase and coalesce resulting in large areas of ecchymosis called *purpura fulminans*, a pathognomonic finding in MD. The presence of *purpura fulminans*, and other clinical signs, meets a case classification category in culture-negative patients that assists in identifying cases. As the disease progresses, shock causes the blood pressure to drop precipitously, and cardiopulmonary arrest ensues. In fatal cases, who underwent autopsy, the finding of hemorrhagic adrenal glands is another way the diagnosis of MD is made. Hemorrhagic adrenal glands in a person with the symptoms of bacterial sepsis is known as Waterhouse-Friderichsen syndrome.

In 2005, approximately a quarter of cases didn't have a positive culture. Without a culture, we could not identify the serogroup or compare bacterial DNA to learn if cases were related. Adding to the undercount are people who die before accessing healthcare and aren't suspected of having MD. These limitations undoubtedly resulted in an undercount of cases and slowness to recognize clusters. Disease surveillance is never perfect, but we rely upon it to detect unusual patterns of disease. Fortunately, in 2006, when MD cases were beginning to pile up, we got an offer from our Wadsworth Center laboratory colleagues. They had developed a PCR test for *N. meningitidis* and were willing to test culture-negative patients. Not only did the test detect if *N. meningitidis* was present, but also the serogroup. This was a huge help and allowed us to presumptively link cases to the burgeoning outbreak.

Paula was one of the MD investigators. She grew up on the Lower East Side and was a lifelong New Yorker. She had been married to a police officer and approached her work with no less diligence than a homicide detective. MD is a social disease. It's transmitted during close and prolonged contact. Paula knew that patients, if they were well enough to speak with us, often withheld vital information. Over repeated interviews, Paula would extract the information we needed to implement control measures. Eventually, she learned that the two cases who briefly shared an apartment also shared drugs. As new cases came in, we inquired about drug use. Some were recovered addicts or in methadone programs. Others reported family members with addiction. Most of the MD patients had some link to Central Brooklyn communities.

The outbreak smoldered. Three cases in January, two in February and March, five in April, then one in May. We gave antibiotic prophylaxis to the contacts of cases, but they weren't the ones getting sick. The disease was spreading in the community and was finding susceptible individuals. We sent health alerts but by the end of May there had been seventeen cases and five deaths. We pushed for a targeted vaccination campaign, but the CDC was lukewarm to the idea, and our immunization program voted against it. The concern was that it would be too difficult to target the at-risk population and even if we could, we didn't have much of a chance to convince enough people at risk to get vaccinated. Overall, their main objection was that it wouldn't be effective. In reality, there was very little data on the effectiveness of community vaccination to control MD outbreaks. Vaccines have mostly been used in closed groups, such as schools where all the members are known. We didn't know what proportion needed to be vaccinated to stop the outbreak. To control a disease like measles you need to reach 90% or better community immunity. MD is not nearly as contagious as measles, but the level of immunity needed to stop an outbreak was unknown.

In early June we were notified about a new case. The forty-six-year-old woman lived in an apartment building in the Bedford-Stuyvesant neighborhood of Brooklyn and had died from meningococcemia. She was now case number twenty-one of the outbreak. But before we could absorb this news, three additional cases were reported the same evening. All three lived in the same apartment complex as the forty-six-year-old woman and were either part of her extended family or a close contact.

While the PHNs worked to identify close contacts in need of antibiotic prophylaxis, I attended a hastily convened town hall meeting at the apartment complex. The meeting was held in a basement recreation room and the mood was tense. In situations such as this, people don't want to hear scientific details or probabilities. They want to know what they need to do to protect themselves and their families. I kept my comments brief, a summary of what we knew and what we were doing and moved on to take questions. We had decided to broaden our prophylaxis criteria because we couldn't easily identify who had contact with the family. We brought antibiotics with us to facilitate close-contact prophylaxis and stayed until there were no more questions. I was asked about early signs and what to do if a child has a fever. There were concerns about common spaces and the elevators which I did my best to dispel as risk factors. They were anxious, but no one was angry.

Before I became a D⊗D I was a pediatrician on a mobile medical unit treating children living in homeless shelters. One of those shelters was a few blocks from the apartment complex in Brooklyn where the four MD cases had occurred. The mobile unit was a bus that was reconfigured to have a waiting area, nursing station, vaccination cubicle, and two exam rooms. We were parked out front one fall afternoon as dusk approached. I was in the side exam room writing my note on the last patient of the day when I heard a thud. We kept cans of infant formula in the cabinet so I figured a can must have fallen. I went out to look and found a round hole in the cabinet door in the rear exam room. The hole was about four feet from the floor. I walked the length of the aisle through the waiting area to the front of the bus where the nurse was standing and staring at the windshield. Moments earlier she had been sitting on the dashboard. Just above where her shoulder had been, was a neatly pierced hole in the glass left by a bullet. The police thought someone had used the van for target practice calling it a random act, not unlike how MD was moving through the community.

After the building cluster, we were more insistent that the department needed to offer vaccine to the affected community. Using data from the NYS Office of Addiction Services and Supports, we estimated that the target population of current and former recreational drug users and their household contacts in four Central Brooklyn zip codes was approximately 10,000. We convinced our health commissioner of the urgent need to implement a vaccine campaign and with the help of community-based organizations and nurses on furlough from the school health program, we established vaccine clinics throughout the affected Brooklyn neighborhoods. Active or former recreational drug users, and their close contacts, were advised to get vaccinated. Vaccination sites used existing health centers, methadone treatment centers, homeless shelters, syringe exchange programs, residential drug treatment facilities, soup kitchens, and correctional facilities. The vaccine campaign ran from late June to the end of August and vaccinated 2,763 people.

How recreational drugs figured into MD transmission wasn't clear. Close contact was likely a factor as could be the sharing of drug paraphernalia. A similar outbreak of MD occurred in Florida in the late 1990s and was linked to a social network of marijuana users.[50] In the NYC outbreak, some cases were current recreational drug users of marijuana, cocaine, including crack cocaine, or heroin. While others were in drug treatment programs or had contact with drug users, suggesting that there was another level of social component to outbreak transmission. Two MD cases connected to the outbreak occurred after the vaccine campaign, one in September and one in November 2006. The final outbreak-associated case count was twenty-three with seven deaths. Overall, the citywide MD case count for 2006 was elevated at fifty-nine cases, the most since 1999. Whether the vaccine campaign ended the outbreak, or it burned out on its own we'll never know. MD the serial killer had retreated into the shadows.

The more I learned about MD, the more I kept returning to something my mother had told me as a child about my paternal grandfather, Papa Jack. Jacob J. Weiss was born in Brooklyn on April 18, 1893, to immigrants from Ukraine who left their homeland to escape pogroms. He was the second of five children and his father, my great-grandfather, built houses in Brooklyn. After graduating from NYU Medical School in 1915 he completed an internship and worked as a clinical assistant at Columbia University Medical School. He then registered for the Army and was sent to France during the final months of World War I. After the war, he was a general practitioner in the Bronx for nearly forty years but was forced to retire due to hearing loss. Papa Jack spent his retirement taking long walks on the Grand Concourse. He'd buy the daily paper for a nickel, sit on a park bench, and read. Out of courtesy, he'd occasionally treat an old patient.

I have no direct memories of Papa Jack. He died before my second birthday. I know him only through black-and-white photos and items handed down to me by my father. In one photo, Jack is a tall, dignified figure, leaning against the mantle in his apartment. He is wearing a suit and sporting round, tortoiseshell glasses, his brown hair is parted in the middle, and he has a thin mustache in the style of Errol Flynn and John Barrymore. In his hand is a pipe. In another photograph, he sat at his desk adorned with a black, rotary phone and a microscope. The Bronx apartment where he lived was on the Grand Concourse at the intersection of 161st Street. My grandmother continued to live there after Papa Jack's death and kept the apartment dark and filled with overstuffed Victorian furniture. The glass bowls on the coffee table were filled with fruit-filled hard candies that no matter how many times I sampled them, tasted awful. I learned how to play card games like casino and poker from my grandmother in that apartment and inherited Papa Jack's Dictaphone, a device that recorded his patient notes onto green plastic disks, and his wire-rimmed sunglasses, pocket watch, and microscope. I broke the watch, lost the sunglasses, and used every disk to record music from a transistor radio. "Cecilia," by Simon and Garfunkel, was one of the songs I recorded. It reminded me of my grandmother whose name was Ceil. The microscope I think is still in my brother's basement. What kept popping into my head was my mother's words that Papa Jack would have lived if they had only given him sulfur.

For my eighth birthday, I received a chemistry set, and in it was a square, glass bottle of yellow sulfur powder. I recall wondering why I had access to the stuff when it wasn't there for my grandfather when he needed it. What I heard as sulfur was really "sulfa," an abbreviation for the antibiotic sulfonamide, which was used in the 1950s to treat bacterial infections. My father knew very little about what killed his father, and my mother died in 1980, before I went to medical school. The mystery would remain.

In 2007, there were twenty-two MD cases in NYC, the fewest number of cases ever. The following year there were twenty-eight. This continued a trend that had begun prior to the outbreak. I wondered why. I knew that vaccines had dramatically reduced the incidence of several communicable diseases, such as polio, measles, and more recently *Haemophilus influenzae*. However, they had all benefited from being included in childhood vaccination recommendations; MD was not.

As part of the declining trend in MD in NYC was an increase in the age of cases and a near disappearance of serogroup B in young children. Fewer child cases explained the increase in the median age of cases, but why were fewer children getting MD? It turned out that one of the *H. influenzae* vaccines on the market utilized an outer membrane protein from *N. meningitidis* serogroup B. Could the *H. influenzae* vaccine inadvertently be providing children immunity to MD? We alerted the manufacturer to our findings and theory. It took several years and reminders before they dug into banked blood from vaccine trials in South America. When they finally got back to us, they couldn't find proof that the vaccine produced any measurable immunity to MD.

Just like I haven't forgotten about Ethel, there was an MD case from 2009 that has stayed with me. Roxanne was a seventeen-year-old at a Lower Manhattan high school. She was an athlete, a member of the choir and theater club, and drew comics for the school newspaper. One week after New Year's, Roxanne developed a headache, fever, and body aches. She died the next day. MD, the serial killer, had taken another life. Many thousands of teenagers experience these symptoms every winter. While very few of them have MD, the statistic is of little consolation to friends and family members. MD can be a swift killer and there is a point of no return where antibiotics and life support cannot intervene. Patients may appear well enough, but there are usually telltale signs. Severe muscle pain and elevated heart rate are two common ones as is a rapidly developing rash. Lab tests also reveal elevated white blood cell counts and decreased platelets. Roxanne was a vibrant seventeen-year-old. A young woman with talents in poetry, music, and art. A person who genuinely cared about others. All who knew her looked forward to seeing the good she would add to the world. Her death was a staggering loss to the community. Parents should not have to bury their children.

Where had Roxanne encountered MD? At school? When she visited a sick friend in the hospital? In the East Village where she'd go to hear music? Some questions have no answers. One answer we were able to give her family was that the perpetrator was *N. meningitidis* serogroup B. Meningococcal vaccine at the time was recommended prior to college entrance, but it wouldn't have protected her against serogroup B.

In August of 2010, MD struck again. The victim was a middle-aged, HIV-infected, gay man from Manhattan, who died soon after presenting to the emergency department. He had a sore throat, headache, fever, and a rash for two days. Identifying close contacts focused on household contacts including sexual contacts. Paula identified three close contacts, but something nagged at her, and she kept digging. Through the man's longtime partner, Paula obtained the numbers dialed from his cell phone in the week before the illness onset. She worked her way down the list of numbers and spoke to a man who disclosed that the decedent had, unbeknownst to his partner, been using an online app to meet men for sex. With the help of colleagues in the Sexually Transmitted Infections (STI) Bureau, we reached out to the operator of the app and sent out messages to users the decedent had contacted. The message alerted them to their possible exposure to MD. One person responded and was offered antibiotic prophylaxis. Others may have opted to consult with their physicians for prophylaxis rather than the government. Paula also uncovered that the decedent had been sharing drugs and she identified another contact needing antibiotic prophylaxis. It came as little surprise that when the DNA analysis of the *N. meningitidis* isolate returned a week later it was a PFGE match to the 2006 outbreak strain pattern.

I kept returning to the question of what my mother had meant when she said Papa Jack would have been saved by sulfa. By 1959, sulfa had been replaced by newer and better antibiotics, but the drug was still an option for MD prophylaxis. Was this a clue to what had caused my grandfather's death? Had he been exposed to MD? I contacted a friend in the Office of Vital Statistics, and she explained how to find a death certificate. It took several months— even bureaucracy for bureaucrats is slow. Papa Jack died on April 21, 1959, three days after his sixty-sixth birthday, which per my cousin Nancy, was celebrated with a party. Could an exposure to MD have happened at his birthday party?

Papa Jack had been taken to the Bronx hospital near his home. The same hospital where he had practiced and I was born. The immediate cause of death was toxemia due to overwhelming bacterial infection. He was also diagnosed with pneumonia, but the clue I had been searching for was on the last line of the death certificate. In Part II, under other significant conditions, was listed

Waterhouse-Friderichsen Syndrome. There had been an autopsy and infarction of the adrenal glands was noted. My grandfather had been a victim of MD.

The doctor who signed the certificate was Henry White. I located a Dr. White, retired and living in California. I called, introduced myself to his wife, and asked if Dr. White had ever worked in the Bronx. He had. She passed the phone to her husband. I explained the strange coincidence that led me to call. That as the NYC epidemiologist responsible for meningococcal disease control I had learned that the disease had felled my grandfather, who had been a physician. I asked Dr. White what he recalled about MD when he was in training. Were there many cases? Was testing available? Did he recall if there had been an outbreak in the Bronx? What antibiotics were available to him? Dr. White was cordial, but he couldn't remember.

The next chapter in the MD saga began in 2011. Laura Miller was in her last semester of graduate school at the Columbia Mailman School of Public Health. She wanted to get experience in infectious diseases as her career goal was to work internationally, so she applied for an internship with the D✪Ds. The internship I administered was designed for first-year graduate students and was to last eighteen months. Laura had less than six months before she would graduate. It didn't seem like a good fit. Bright, energetic, and enthusiastic, Laura had completed classwork that would be valuable for research projects, but I already had selected two first-year student candidates. I had long wanted to analyze all the MD data we had collected from the previous decades but there was a catch. The data was all on paper and many of the case investigations had been sent to storage. Laura was willing to tackle the project, so along with her fellow interns Arianne Ramautar and Lola Arakaki, they combed through the files, extracted data, and meticulously entered it all into a database.

We matched the data to the death and HIV registries. It was slow and tedious work. We waited for files to arrive from storage. There were missing case files and data points and illegible handwriting. We also had to deal with the limitations of lab testing. Although Laura was about to graduate, and she didn't need the project to meet her curriculum requirements, she kept at it. One early evening when I was on my way to the gym, she called me from the office. Excitedly, she had a finding she wanted to review. I had expected we'd find an increased risk of death in HIV-infected individuals, but that wasn't what Laura was calling about. She was a bit out of breath as if she just ran to catch the subway and relayed that she had found a large relative risk. The relative risk is a measure of association that compares disease among populations. Persons living with HIV or AIDS had a ten-fold increased risk of contracting MD compared to HIV-uninfected people. Ten-fold? In epidemiological studies, a two- or three-fold increase in risk is newsworthy, and often drug companies will tout drugs that provide a 30% improvement which is equivalent to a relative risk of 1.3. A relative risk of ten was big news.

We checked Laura's code and math. It was correct. We located a recent research study from South Africa published in June 2010 which found a comparable risk ratio.[51] We notified the CDC and urged them to add HIV infection to the list of meningococcal vaccine recommendations. It took two years of calls and meetings, and the events described below, before the Advisory Committee on Immunization Practices agreed to add people infected with HIV to the list of groups recommended to receive meningococcal vaccination. Laura's ground-breaking research was published online in the *Annals of Internal Medicine* in October 2013.[52]

While the wheels of public health policy ground slowly

forward, we had another MD problem. Six cases occurred in a three-week period at the end of December 2010 and the beginning of January 2011 and three people died. The NYC Health Code requires that MD be reported immediately upon suspicion or diagnosis. The reason is that the administration of antibiotic prophylaxis is most effective when done quickly. Unfortunately, as happened before, several of the cases were not reported promptly. Three of the six cases were serogroup C, and one was indistinguishable by PFGE to the 2006 outbreak strain. The sixth case of the cluster that occurred in January 2011 was in an HIV-uninfected, gay man.

The first half of 2011 was typical for MD. There were six cases in January, zero in February, four in March, one in April, and two each in May and June. Summer months don't usually have many cases but there was one in July and then, in August, MD stepped out of character as it struck three cases, all who were gay men. The cases occurred within days of each other, and they all lived in different boroughs. One was Black, one Latinx, and the other was White. One was HIV-infected. No social connection among the men could be ascertained. When the PHL shared the *N. meningitidis* DNA analysis we were a bit puzzled. Only two could be analyzed and neither DNA pattern was a PFGE match to the 2006 outbreak strain. But the patterns were close. Ever changing, MD was adapting.

We looked back in our database and made phone calls to patients to fill in gaps in sexual orientation. In the nine years from 2001–2009, there were nine cases of MD in gay men, about one per year. Three in a single month was unusual. In the absence of a link to a discrete community, there wasn't support for a vaccination effort as we had done in 2006.

Our colleagues in STI educated us on the use of drugs in

the gay community—cocaine, ketamine, ecstasy, amyl nitrate, and gamma-hydroxybutyrate, among others. Drug use was a plausible explanation for how MD had entered the gay community. We had just discovered the link between HIV and MD and were terrified by the havoc the disease could cause in an immunocompromised community. In the remaining months of 2011, there were ten MD cases, only one was caused by serogroup C, a thirty-five-year-old man who denied being gay. Two cases had unknown serogroups, and they were both women. It would prove to be a temporary reprieve.

New Year's Eve 2011 brought about the end of an eventful year that saw a nuclear disaster in Japan, Hurricane Irene, emerging effects of global warming throughout the American South and Midwest, the death of Osama bin Laden, and the shooting of Arizona Senator Gabby Giffords. MD didn't wait long to make its mark on the new year. On January 17, a twenty-three-year-old gay man with HIV arrived at a Brooklyn emergency department breathing fast—30 respirations per minute—and with a heart rate of 165 beats per minute. A normal, resting heart rate for his age is in the range of 60 to 75 beats per minute. His temperature was 100.2°F and he complained of a cough, sore throat, and rash. Not long after presenting to the emergency department, he lost consciousness and died. His demise was so rapid that there was no time to administer antibiotics. From his blood was recovered *N. meningitidis*, serogroup C. The hospital failed to report the case for nine days.

I frequently gave talks to the medical community about MD and learned that the reason clinicians didn't report MD cases was that the diagnosis wasn't suspected because the patient didn't have symptoms of meningitis. Meningitis is just one presentation of MD and it's not the most fatal. Meningococcemia, the blood infection that provokes an out-of-control immune response, kills most victims of MD. Meningitis results when bacteria present in the blood cross the blood-brain barrier and enter the spinal fluid. If the patient can clear the infection from the blood, as many do, the patient has only meningitis and survival is better than in patients with meningococcemia.

Another MD case occurred in a twenty-seven-year-old gay man from Brooklyn in March, then a twenty-one-year-old gay man from the Bronx was felled by MD in May. One more in June, this time the fifty-nine-year-old HIV-infected man from Brooklyn who survived. All had serogroup C and had no discernible connection, other than being gay. We asked the Advisory Committee on Immunization Practices during their October 2011 meeting to recommend a meningococcal vaccine for HIV-infected individuals, but they elected to table the issue.

August in NYC is hot and humid. Concrete absorbs the heat and radiates it back at night so sunset doesn't necessarily provide relief. Only living near trees does. Those that can, leave the city for cooler climates—the beach or mountains. Most of the bureau took vacation in August, but I preferred fall vacations when the national parks were less crowded. I was at my desk in late August 2012 when the next MD case occurred. The thirty-one-year-old man was found by a relative confused, unsteady, and combative, with a fever of 102.5°F, during a wellness check. He was diagnosed with MD meningitis, serogroup C, and survived. Unlike the previous 2012 cases in gay men, he confided to Paula that he met men online for sex and used marijuana and crystal meth, but he didn't provide any names so we could alert the contacts and offer prophylaxis. It felt like we had reached a tipping point.

Two days before the ten-year memorial of 9/11 there was another MD case in a forty-two-year-old gay man who also had met sex partners online and used drugs. As one gay man who worked at the health department confided, if they're meeting anonymous sex partners online, we needn't ask about drugs, they're being used. The new case survived and named the previous case as a sexual contact. It highlighted the importance of getting cases to name contacts. If we had known, we could've prevented the latter's illness. Less than two weeks later, at 4:00 p.m. on Friday, we received a call from the Office of the Chief Medical Examiner (OCME).

A thirty-two-year-old man was found unresponsive by his roommate the day before. He was pronounced dead at the scene. This unfortunately is not an unusual circumstance. The early symptoms of MD are not unlike other illnesses. Progression to the point where you can no longer call for help can be rapid. This feature of the disease likely contributes to underreporting of MD because people found dead at home do not regularly get tested. In NYC, it is protocol for the OCME to consider MD and notify us. Depending on how long the person goes undetected and the state of decomposition there may be no blood or spinal fluid samples to test. With the assistance of the Wadsworth Center and OCME, we pioneered the use of vitreous humor PCR testing to make the MD diagnoses. Vitreous humor is a thick liquid that fills and maintains the shape of the eyeball. Vitreous humor is in contact with the retinal nerve and thus the central nervous system where MD infections occur. We reasoned that vitreous humor might show evidence of *N. meningitidis* infection. Two of the 2012 outbreak cases were diagnosed using vitreous humor.

In the thirty-two-year-old, the medical examiner was able to obtain spinal fluid and found evidence of meningitis as well as a petechial rash during autopsy. The spinal fluid was positive for *N. meningitidis*. The man was known to be HIV-infected and had multiple male sexual partners; some he met on dating apps. The PHNs got busy trying to identify and notify contacts, a bigger challenge now since they couldn't interview the patient.

Four days later we had another case, number thirteen in the growing MD outbreak among gay men in NYC. He had meningitis, admitted to drug use, but denied meeting men online. He thankfully recovered and offered a new clue. Before getting ill he had attended a birthday celebration at a gay bar in Brooklyn. The same bar had been named by another case. Three of the four cases from August and September—one had a negative culture—had the same strain of serogroup C and all were HIV-infected.

To convince the administration of the need to implement a vaccine campaign, I did the math, convinced that data would demonstrate the extent of the problem and justify spending public resources to ameliorate it. One would think that thirteen cases of MD in gay men would be enough to justify offering vaccination, but the same issues that delayed the vaccine campaign in 2006 were raised. Who precisely is the population at risk? Is the rate elevated? What is the level of risk? Can we focus on a target population? The population estimate of gay men in NYC was 103,000, a seemingly low number, but it was all we had at the time. Comparing the number of MD cases in gay men between the ages of 18-64 to the rest of the male population of the same age range yielded a fifty-three-fold increased MD risk. What's more, the increased MD risk was close to ninety-fold for HIV-infected gay men. Even if the population estimate for gay men was off by a factor of two, or even four, the MD risk was still tremendously elevated. The data compelled the health department to act. On October 4, 2012, the department issued 2012 Health Alert #28 to the medical community recommending that meningococcal vaccine be given to:

> *HIV-infected men who are NYC residents and who had intimate contact with a man met either through an online website, digital application ("app"), or at a bar or party since September 1, 2012.*[53]

The recommendation was more limited than I had hoped, but it was a start. I understood the immunization program's concern about supply and distribution, but this time instead of operating all the vaccine sites, we could enlist the entire medical community. The media quickly picked up on the story and helped spread the word. Unfortunately, cases kept occurring: two more in November, and neither person was HIV-infected. At the end of November, the vaccine recommendations were expanded:

> *Meningococcal vaccine should now also be offered to men who have sex with men, regardless of HIV status, if they live in specific areas of Brooklyn and report intimate contact with a man met either through an online website, digital application ("app"), or at a bar or party since September 1, 2012.*[54]

The department activated the Incident Command System (ICS) to respond to the outbreak. Molly Kratz, who I would later convince her to join the D🟦Ds, worked in the office of the deputy commissioner for the Division of Disease Control in 2012. She was enlisted to coordinate all the various response efforts—from communication to vaccine—no small task. Free vaccine was made available at nine department sites. Medical providers serving the HIV and gay community were assisted in the purchase and administration of the vaccine, which the NYS Department of Health mandated insurance companies to cover. In addition, a blitz of materials, posters, and palm cards were distributed in the affected communities. Community workers visited subway stops, community centers, churches, and businesses to spread the vaccine message to targeted groups. Online advertisements were purchased on major websites and apps used by men to meet men. The department supported vaccine events at bars, clubs, concerts and parties. Dr. Demetre Daskalakis, who would join the department in a few years, volunteered to administer vaccine in bars. Providers were kept informed by a series of health alerts and the media was encouraged to champion the campaign. Coverage by *The New York Times* in March of 2013 provided a much-needed boost to the campaign. Tracking the exact number of doses given was challenging. Large providers submitted a weekly total, but the numbers didn't include all providers. The estimate of vaccine uptake was over 20,000 doses.

After a cluster of four cases and two deaths in late January and February 2013, the vaccine recommendations were further expanded and simplified: (a) All HIV-infected men who have sex with men (MSM); (b) MSM, regardless of HIV status, who regularly have close or intimate contact with men met through an online website, digital application ("app"), or at a bar or party.

I still didn't think the recommendations went far enough. What about HIV-infected women? Non-gay men with HIV? Fortunately, there were no cases in gay men from March 2013 to March 2014, and the outbreak was declared over. All told, MD had infected twenty-two gay men and killed seven of them. Five of the seven who died were HIV-infected. The outbreak was again centered in Brooklyn and primarily affected men of color. Eleven of the cases were African American and four were Latinx. Two women were identified with the same MD strain during 2011–2013. Neither was HIV-infected, and we could not determine how they got exposed to MD. The strain was now in the LGBTQ community, and it was puzzling how it had remained relatively contained within the gay community.

We theorized that similar to its cousin, *Neisseria gonorrhoeae*, MD had gained the ability to survive in the genitourinary tract and perhaps even the colon. Ever the chameleon, this would explain why the strain remained within the gay community. It was being transmitted sexually. To investigate this theory, we designed a carriage study to measure how often the *N. meningitidis* could be found in these anatomical locations in gay men. But before we could start, MD resurfaced.

There was another case involving a gay man in June 2014, followed by three more cases in late August and early September. All were HIV-infected and two had reportedly received two doses of vaccine. The demographics and geography of the latter three cases was highly suggestive that they were part of a social network, however, interviews did not reveal links despite the DNA analysis linking the cases to each other and the MSM serogroup C outbreak strain. Learning if the cases had social links mattered because if the three had contact with each other there was a chance that the MD strain wasn't widely distributed in the community and another outbreak could be averted. We obtained, through voluntary submission and subpoena, cell phone records for the three cases. Kristen Lee, a D❂D with expertise in computer coding, wrote a program to search for any cell phone numbers in all three files. She got a hit. Upon further questioning, it was determined that the three men had all attended the same party. The media picked up on the story and Molly renewed her vaccine outreach efforts.

MD cases in gay men in other parts of the United States and the world were being recognized. There was a cluster in Los Angeles and single cases in Pennsylvania, New Jersey, and Arizona.

Cases were also found in France and Germany, and we were asked to participate in international conference calls to compare notes, review data methods, and share approaches to prevention. The meningococcal carriage study in gay and transexual men was completed in 2017. While the overall carriage rate of any strain of *N. meningitidis* was 23%, we found limited carriage (<1%) in the rectum and urethra. What's more, the 2010–2013 outbreak strain wasn't found. Was the study too late? Or was our theory of sexual transmission wrong?

N. meningitidis keeps changing. An invasive serogroup C strain lost an important capsule gene becoming unencapsulated. While this change might be seen as beneficial as the strain lost the ability to cause severe disease, it gained the ability to better attach to mucosal surfaces, like the lining of the rectum and urethra—a trait found in *N. gonorrhoeae*. The strain next picked up genes from *N. gonorrhoeae* that allowed it to survive in low-oxygen environments, such as the genitourinary tract. This strain began causing urethritis in non-gay men and has moved about the globe.[55,56] The most recent adaptation has been the acquisition of an antimicrobial resistance gene from *N. gonorrhoeae*.[57]

Yvonne Ardan Faur was born in Romania in 1916 and earned a medical degree from the University of Bucharest in 1940, the same year that her country aligned itself with Nazi Germany. She survived World War II and the Holocaust and became the chief microbiologist at Cantacuzino Institute. In 1962, she immigrated to the United States and became a naturalized citizen. She worked at the PHL, received a patent for inventing "NYC media" to better grow *N. meningitidis* and had the bacterium *Roseomonas fauriae* named for her to credit her work characterizing the pink-pigment producing organism. In 1975, Dr. Faur and PHL colleagues noticed something unusual coming from the City's STI clinics.

During a four-month period they found thirty-two patients with
N. meningitidis from the male anal canal, urethra, or female cervix.
Twenty-five patients were males and serogroup B (n=9) was the
most common followed by C (n=8)[58]. Molecular characterization
wasn't possible in 1975 so whether this strain had mutations similar to the current trends is unknown. Dr. Faur was still at PHL
as a consultant when I joined the department in 2000. We briefly
met once, but I did not get the chance to know her before her
death in 2007.

The genetic adaptations of *N. meningitidis* again suggested
the possible expansion of its niche to include sexual transmission.
Colonization of the female reproductive tract could result in neonatal infections. In August 2017, we were alerted about a Bronx
newborn who contracted conjunctivitis on the third day of life.
The routine use of antibiotic eye drops in newborns was implemented to prevent gonorrhea infections. The conjunctivitis turned
out to be caused by *N. meningitidis* and found to be related to a
new strain with borrowed genes from *N. gonorrhoeae*.[59] The child
recovered. A second case of neonatal *N. meningitidis* conjunctivitis occurred in 2021. The D❂Ds remain on alert for additional
cases, including severe disease.

While serogroup C was circulating and attacking the gay
community, serogroup B had set its sights on another subset of the
population: college students. The CDC analyzed MD surveillance
data from 1998–2000 and discovered that college students, specifically freshman living in dormitories, were at an increased risk
of MD. This led them in 2005 to recommend the MenACWY
vaccine for incoming high school and college students. A couple of years later in 2008, an outbreak of serogroup B began on
the campus of Ohio University. Thirteen cases and one death
occurred. Risk factors for infections included kissing more than

one person and membership in a fraternity or sorority.[60] In the six-year period from 2013–2018, the CDC was informed about ten outbreaks on college campuses totaling thirty-nine cases with two deaths.[61] In 2015, the first serogroup B vaccine was licensed in the United States. While the Advisory Committee on Immunization Practices didn't add it to the routine vaccine schedule, they recommended persons 16–23 years of age discuss the need and value of vaccine with their medical provider.

In late January of 2019, an international graduate student returned to Columbia University's campus. Ten days later he presented to health services with fever, severe headache, and vomiting. The student was diagnosed with MD caused by serogroup B. Three days later, a second student from the same graduate program became ill and was also diagnosed with serogroup B MD. Although the two students knew of each other they could not recall anything more than brief, casual hallway conversations. However, their social groups overlapped. We expanded antibiotic prophylaxis to eliminate the organism from individuals in the program who might be carriers. The university responded by offering vaccine to students in the same graduate program. There was no third case.

During my tenure as a D❂D, the number of MD cases in the city steadily declined. The decade 1990–1999 saw approximately fifty cases per year. The decade 2000–2009 had between thirty and forty cases per year. And the following decade, between ten to twenty cases per year. The most reasonable explanation is vaccine. The polysaccharide vaccine was approved in 1985 and was only recommended for adults with risk factors so presumably was not widely used. As opposed to a disease like measles, which requires vaccine coverage > 90% to prevent breakthrough cases, MD has a much lower threshold. The exact value isn't known, but if the polysaccharide vaccine was administered to those at greatest risk for MD could it have contributed to the decline in the 1990s? The timing fits. Most epidemiologists would rightfully be skeptical.

One of the most notable vaccine success stories is *Haemophilus influenzae* type B (Hib, see graph). The disease affects infants and young children causing meningitis, pneumonia, and the very scary epiglottis. Polysaccharide vaccine for Hib was used 1985–1989. When a conjugate vaccine for Hib was approved and put into use beginning in 1989, cases of Hib plummeted.

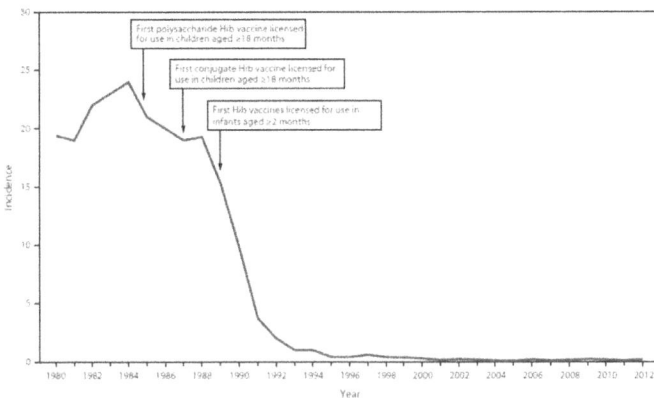

Sources: 1980-1997: National Bacterial Meningitis Reporting System and National Notifiable Diseases Surveillance (NNDSS) data; Adams WG, Deaver KA, Cochi SL, et al. Decline of childhood *Haemophilus influenzae* Type b (Hib) disease in the Hib vaccine era. JAMA 1993;269:221–6; CDC. Progress toward elimination of *Haemophilus influenzae* type b disease among infants and children—United States, 1987-1995. MMWR 1996;45:901–6; CDC. Progress toward elimination of *Haemophilus influenzae* type b disease among infants and children—United States, 1987-1997. MMWR 1998;47:993–8. 1998-2009: NNDSS and Active Bacterial Core Surveillance (ABCs) data. 2010-2012: ABCs cases estimated to the U.S. population.

* Per 100,000 population.

US Incidence of Haemophilus influenzae, Type B Disease, 1980–2012[62]

As mentioned previously, one of the Hib vaccines, PRP-OMP, utilizes as an adjuvant—immune system stimulant—an outer membrane protein from *N. meningitidis* serogroup B. It was approved in 1990 but had competition from other products. We noted a decline in serogroup B in children <1 and between the ages of one and four, the predominant strain affecting these age groups beginning in the early 1990s.

From our Immunization Bureau colleagues we learned the

proportion of PRP-OMP distributed through the Vaccine for Children (VFC) program which provides free vaccine to both private and public providers. Interestingly, the percent of PRP-OMP vaccine distributed to VFC providers in NYC increased from 1995–2000 as follows: 19%, 10%, 26%, 58%, 41%, 58%, respectively. It's not a publishable association data but remains a curious finding.

YEARS	NYC SEROGROUP B, AGES 0-4 YEARS
1989-1991	28
1992-1994	16
1995-1997	13
1999-2000	6
2001-2002	1

Incidence of Serogroup B Meningococcal Disease in Children 0–4 Years

When the newer, more effective MD conjugate vaccines were added to the routine childhood vaccination schedule—first for adolescents between the ages of eleven and eighteen, then for children between the ages of two and ten at increased risk in 2007, and then as a routine recommendation for infants in 2020—the decline in MD case counts accelerated, reaching the lowest point in surveillance history during the COVID-19 pandemic. Not surprising as MD is a social disease, and with people staying at home, there was less opportunity to become exposed to a carrier. Case counts have rebounded somewhat, and as I write this, two MD situations have emerged.

The CDC announced in March 2024 that there has been an increase in MD throughout the United States caused by sero-group Y. The MD case counts in the first quarter of 2024 went from eighty-one in 2023 to 142 in 2024. Cases characteristics are now thirty to sixty years of age and overwhelmingly African Americans. The proportion of HIV-infected is also high at 15%.[63] No mention was made in the CDC alert about cases among gay men, but nearly two-thirds of the cases have been male. *N. meningitidis* resistance to ciprofloxacin, the most common drug used for prophylaxis, has increased in NYC necessitating a switch to other antibiotics. These two situations together fit with the adaptation of MD as a sexually transmitted disease. *N. gonorrhoeae* developed resistance to ciprofloxacin early this century. While vaccine has curtailed MD's serial killer reign, the bacterium continues to evolve and find new niches.

I feel like a retired detective with unfinished business. I suppose in a way I am, but the feeling goes deeper. And not just any detective, but the ones you see on *Dateline* or *48 Hours*. The detective who worked for decades on that one egregious, unsolved case trying to bring closure to a family whose loved one was murdered. Meningococcal disease is still out there. Contemplating its next move, jumping from person-to-person, until it finds the next susceptible host.

CHAPTER 9

Bandits in the Park

The first sign of trouble was an email attachment with a virus. Sally Slavinski, the BCD's public health veterinarian, received the email on August 27, 2009. The attachment wasn't a computer virus but a real one, a report of animal rabies. The positive test was from a raccoon, not unusual as raccoons are the most prevalent rabid species found in NYC. What was unusual was the location—Manhattan, specifically the north end of Central Park—one of the most popular tourist destinations in the world attracting 25 million visitors each year.

Rabid raccoons were routinely found in the Bronx and Staten Island but infrequently in Manhattan. People were known to move raccoons found on their property, and it was chalked up to illegal translocation. Sally alerted staff and called her colleague Richard Simon at the NYC Parks Department. They considered the implications and commiserated. The NY State and City health laws require dogs, as well as cats, to be vaccinated against rabies with booster shots every one to three years to maintain immunity. But Sally and Richard knew that many pet owners don't remember, don't bother, or can't afford to vaccinate. New Yorkers are allowed to let their dogs run free in parks at certain times of the day where an unvaccinated dog might encounter a rabid raccoon. The dog would have to be put down or placed in six-month quarantine at a cost to the owner. Both prospects Sally did not relish. But there was reason for optimism. It had been more than fifty years since the last case of dog rabies in NYC.

Sally and Richard decided to increase the level of rabid animal surveillance which was already high by public health standards. Many jurisdictions only test raccoons if involved in an encounter with humans or pets to advise post-exposure prophylaxis (PEP) decisions. It is a cost-saving measure. The NYC protocol included testing raccoons found injured or with neurologic symptoms. The protocol provided critical surveillance data so the magnitude and geography of rabies could be tracked. Sally and Richard optimistically agreed the rabid raccoon found at the north end of the park was likely an illegal translocation, but they increased awareness among park rangers and added any raccoon found dead to the testing algorithm. Sally then entered the result in the surveillance database and took a deep breath.

Rabies is a virus uniquely adapted to mammals. In particular skunks, foxes, raccoons, and numerous species of bats. It is a bullet-shaped virus and consists of a single strand of ribonucleic acid (RNA). The virus usually spreads to humans from an infected animal through contact with saliva either from a bite or the introduction into an open wound or mucous membrane. After a period of quiescence, the rabies virus begins its slow trek to the brain along peripheral nerves. The disease in humans is nearly universally fatal once symptoms begin which can occur anytime from several weeks to many months after the exposure. This is why PEP is given soon after the exposure. PEP is most effective if given before the virus enters the peripheral nerves. The greater the amount of virus present in the animal's saliva, the more numerous the bite wounds, and their proximity to the brain, the shorter the time available to prevent infection.

Rabid animals lose interest in food and grooming and behave as if confused. Nocturnal creatures come out during the day and wander beyond the boundaries of their normal habitat to encounter domestic animals and humans. While the image of a rabid animal is one of excessive aggression this is not the most common behavior change. Most animals become listless and retreat to their dens. They suffer from progressive muscle paralysis, difficulty breathing, and die within a week of symptom onset. In humans, the pathology is very much the same. The virus travels along nerves to the brain where it causes encephalitis, progressive deterioration of nervous function, and death. Paralysis of the swallowing muscles gives rise to hydrophobia, the fear of choking on water, the former name for human rabies. No case of rabies has been documented from a human bite, but the virus can be found in the human salivary glands and human-to-human transmission has been reported in countries outside the United States.

Rabies in America was first recognized in terrestrial animals at the beginning of the eighteenth century. It is believed to have come west with domesticated dogs. Throughout the eighteenth and nineteenth centuries, most rabies exposures to humans were from dogs or livestock. As pet vaccination programs expanded after World War II and surveillance improved, wild animal rabies surpassed domestic as the leading cause. Today, the species most tested and found rabid in the United States is the raccoon, while human rabies cases are linked to bats.

In 1994, a fourteen-year-old boy from Texas died of rabies. His illness began with a sore throat and trouble breathing and was followed by unusual behavior that fluctuated between inactivity and hyperactivity. He died two weeks after onset. He was infected with a dog strain of rabies, but no exposure could be found other than to a sick puppy. The puppy died two months before his illness and was unavailable for testing, but its mother and littermates were all well. Three years earlier a woman, also from Texas, died from canine rabies. She too had no discernible exposure. Rabid animals in proximity to humans are a bad outcome waiting to happen.

The rest of the summer and fall of 2009 were relatively quiet. At the south end of Central Park, several dead raccoons were found but they all tested negative for rabies. It was still possible they were incubating rabies and succumbed to wounds inflicted by a rabid raccoon. Testing only picks up the virus once it reaches the brain, a process that can take from days to weeks in wild animals. If the dead raccoons had been infected, at least they couldn't have infected others.

On December 1, the other raccoon dropped. The day after Thanksgiving, near the tennis house in Central Park, two raccoons were found, —one injured, the other dead. Because of the holiday they weren't tested until the following week and the results came to Sally that Tuesday. The injured raccoon was negative but the dead one tested positive. She was devastated. She had little time to prevent rabies from establishing itself in the world's most popular park. Sally wasn't exactly envisioning rabid dogs running through the streets of New York nipping at joggers and nannies, but the second positive raccoon in Central Park was quite disconcerting. Eerily, the news came on the same day when in 1885 a rabid dog ran through nearby streets. It happened in the early morning hours across the river in Newark, New Jersey. Children were on their way to school. Six were attacked, and four incurred bites, the equivalent of a death sentence. A local physician, who had read about Louis Pasteur's success with a rabies vaccine just months before, placed an editorial in the local paper. He implored that money be raised to send these financially poor and most unfortunate children to Paris. He sent a cable across the ocean and Pasteur agreed to treat them. The community responded and raised the money needed to send the four boys across the Atlantic Ocean. They were the first Americans to receive Pasteur's vaccine. They arrived in time and all four survived.[64]

Louis Pasteur was an innovative genius who used his powers of observation to make sense of the biological world. A chemist with no formal training in medicine, he was at the end of his prodigious career when he began to work on rabies. With a vaccine for chicken cholera to his credit and knowledge of Edward Jenner's work with cowpox vaccination to prevent smallpox, Pasteur conceived the idea that rabies could be prevented by administering doses of attenuated virus, a process to make it less virulent. Through a series of laboratory experiments that began in 1881, he infected rabbits with rabies and exposed spinal cord tissue to dry air for increasing lengths of time. After fourteen days of drying, the rabies virus from the rabbit spinal cord was no longer able to infect dogs yet immunized them against challenges of the virulent strain. Pasteur showed that the treatment worked if given after the occurrence of a rabid animal bite but before symptoms began. The first patient to ever receive rabies post-exposure vaccine was nine-year-old Joseph Meister in 1885. The second person to receive treatment was fifteen-year-old Jean Baptiste Jupille, who was savagely bitten by a rabid dog when he came to the courageous defense of a group of school children in imminent peril. Both boys survived and Meister went on to work at the Pasteur Institute.

Pasteur's discovery led to the practice of rabies PEP which is still the standard of care today. Rabies immune globulin, extracted from the blood of volunteers previously immunized in combination with the rabies vaccine series—now a four-dose schedule—is highly effective in preventing disease when given soon after exposure. The treatment works if the exposed person has an intact immune system and can make antibodies. Sally worried about what would happen if the person bitten had AIDS or cancer or was a transplant recipient on immunosuppressant therapy. Would the person mount a sufficient antibody response to prevent disease or be the first case of human rabies in NYC in over sixty years?

As a kid growing up on Long Island, Sally had pets like most kids. Gerbils, hamsters, and even a rabbit. Sally understood her pets better than she did her classmates, preferring their furry company. Good thing those socially awkward years were well behind her because she'd need all her people skills to obtain the cooperation of city, state, and federal agencies as well as the public's. Wildlife experts advised that there were just two options to interrupt rabies transmission among Central Park raccoons: vaccinate, depopulate, or a combination of the two. While raccoon vaccination was unlikely to draw much opposition, depopulation was a completely different issue. By lowering the raccoon density there would be fewer opportunities for rabid raccoons to encounter and infect well ones, thus slowing and eventually halting the spread. The quickest way to achieve population reduction is by capturing and euthanizing raccoons. Kill a kit and caboodle of raccoons, the well along with the rabid. This would most certainly provoke opposition.

There was enough evidence to show that once established, rabies would be difficult to eradicate from the Central Park raccoon population. The only hope was that it hadn't invaded too far and if they acted quickly there was a chance a full-blown epizootic or animal epidemic could be averted. Sally spoke to an expert in Canada who had dealt with a similar situation a decade earlier. He recommended an immediate raccoon depopulation by 80% followed by trapping and vaccination.

The park is an ideal raccoon habitat. Unlike their upstate cousins who travel as much as five miles a night to find food, raccoons in Central Park have an abundance of food with very few health hazards. Raccoons have few natural predators, and although young raccoons can fall prey to coyotes and foxes, these carnivores are rare in NYC. With slower city speed limits and less need to travel outside of the park, roadkill is also a less frequent phenomenon in NYC. The population of raccoons in Central Park was unknown but estimated to be between 400 and 500. That meant killing upward of 400 raccoons. There was a sense that the population of raccoons in Central Park was increasing. The Parks Department registered an increase in sightings and complaints as well as nuisance calls to the City's 3-1-1 hotline. Then in June 2009, a raccoon made its acting debut at Shakespeare in the Park. During the first act of *Twelfth Night*, a raccoon upstaged actors Anne Hathaway and Audra McDonald by evoking raucous laughs from the audience in an otherwise somber scene.

Sally was going to need help, a lot of help. She drafted an agenda and made a list of agencies to invite to join a Central Park Raccoon Rabies Task Force. The first conference call was set for December 2. On the conference call were colleagues from the department's Bureau of Veterinary Public Health Services, NYC PHL, NYC Parks, Animal Care and Control (ACC), the City's vendor for processing animals for rabies testing, the non-profit Central Park Conservancy (CPC) and the NY Department of Environmental Conservation (DEC). The US Department of Agriculture (USDA), NY Department of Health (NYSDOH), the New York Wadsworth Center, the Wildlife Conservation

Society (WCS), and others from the health department joined later calls. After introductions, Sally summarized the history of raccoon rabies in NYC.

The spread of raccoon rabies in the United States is a story unto itself. It wasn't until 1938 that rabies in animals and humans became nationally notifiable, and cases counted. Although raccoon rabies was found in all states except Hawaii by the 1970s, the occurrences were infrequent and sporadic. Lab techniques to type strains to specific species were not yet available and it was believed that the disease spilled over from other animals and was not established in the raccoon population.

The above epidemiology of raccoon rabies was not true in Florida. The first rabid raccoon there was identified on the east-central coast in 1947. Over the next fifteen years, raccoon rabies spread throughout Florida and across the border into Alabama. Destruction of raccoon habitat forced migration to urban centers and increased their numbers. The denser the human population, the denser the raccoon population became. Rabies followed. Transmission was occurring from raccoon to raccoon and the path of the virus was north. By the late 1970s, the epizootic spread beyond Florida further into Alabama, Georgia, and South Carolina with nearly 500 rabid raccoons identified in 1979. Then something happened to accelerate the northward march of raccoon rabies.

One can characterize the environmental behavior of *Homo sapiens* as act first and consider the consequences later. DDT, the ozone layer depletion, toxic waste sites, and global warming are just a few examples of our environmentally reckless behavior. As the raccoon rabies epizootic was raging in the Southeast, hunters, and perhaps others, moonlighted as raccoon travel agents. Thousands of raccoons were legally and illegally moved from

Florida to Virginia and North Carolina. On at least one occasion a rabid raccoon was documented in a shipment.

In 1977 a single rabid raccoon was found in West Virginia near the Virginia border. The next year three rabid raccoons were found across the border in Virginia. This was followed by a modest twelve rabid raccoons in the Virginias, which increased to twenty-one by 1980. A new epizootic was brewing. By 1982, it bloomed to more than 800 rabid raccoons involving four states and the District of Columbia. The epizootic reached Delaware in 1987 and New Jersey two years later. Moving at a rate of about thirty miles per year, raccoon rabies crossed the border into NYC in 1992.

During the first conference call, Sally explained to the task force that raccoon rabies had become enzootic in the Bronx and Staten Island with an average of seven to ten rabid raccoons per year. About one per year were found in Queens and Manhattan. No rabid raccoons had yet to be found in Brooklyn. She laid out the available options for control: (1) oral rabies vaccine (ORV); (2) cull the raccoon population; (3) trap, injectable vaccination, and release (TVR) or some combination of all three. Whichever they chose, they had to act quickly. Experts looking at the geography and ecology of Central Park assessed that raccoon density was likely to be very high, an ideal setting for rapid transmission and establishment of enzootic rabies.

Sally had a low opinion of oral rabies vaccines. Although they have been employed with success in halting the westward spread of raccoon rabies into Ohio, they hadn't worked very well in her experience or reading of the literature. The percent of raccoons that developed immunity was less than 25% and ORV carries the risk of accidental exposure to pets or humans. ORV utilizes a recombinant rabies protein in a live vaccinia virus vehicle. The bait used is a fragrant fish by-product. Though not a live rabies virus, if eaten by pets or handled by humans it could cause vaccinia. It is perhaps good for inaccessible rural, wooden, or mountainous areas with a low human population density, but most of Central Park seemed like a less-than-ideal location for its use. Sally was mostly concerned that ORV wasn't a good choice for a rapid response as it needed to be dosed regularly over time to have an effect.

Culling, the humane depopulation of raccoons by capturing and euthanasia, was at best controversial. The task force was sure to incur strenuous opposition from animal welfare groups. Wildlife and public health officials in Ontario had made use of culling to halt the spread of raccoon rabies into the Toronto area from northern New York and recommended this approach in concert with TVR. Their experience, however, suggested that culling would need to be a yearly event, at least in the short-term. The ecology of the Canadian-New York border, however, was unlike that of Central Park.

Trapping and vaccinating raccoons was the most attractive option. Accepting the cost and effort it required, it offered much higher immunization rates than ORV and a way to simultaneously enumerate the raccoon population. By tagging vaccinated raccoons, an estimate of the population could be made by comparing the number recaptured to the total. With Sally's leadership, the task force decided on a course of action. It was TVR-based and included culling. It would take weeks to work out the logistics of the plan, but they decided on a set of immediate actions. Notifications were sent to both the veterinary and medical community to alert them to the presence of raccoon rabies in Central Park. A press release from the department notified the public and advised them to vaccinate pets, keep dogs on leashes, and avoid encounters with raccoons. Signs were placed in the park, especially in areas popular with dog owners. Fliers were distributed to area businesses, schools, pet stores, and throughout the mass transit system. Surveillance was increased. Park workers already on alert for sick or dead raccoons would be extra vigilant and private trappers of nuisance raccoons would submit them for testing. They closed the call agreeing to speak again the next day to begin working out the logistics.

Unbeknownst to Sally, as she was on the conference call, a raccoon was on its way to the PHL for testing. It had sores on its face and was found gnawing on its own leg outside of the north gate to the Conservatory Garden at Fifth Avenue and 106th Street. It was not aggressive but became the third rabid raccoon found in Central Park. So far there had not been any *known* rabid raccoon encounters with either dogs or humans. However, there had been a troubling episode that summer involving a woman who had too much to drink and fell asleep in Central Park next to her food on a picnic blanket. The woman awoke to see a raccoon helping itself to her dinner and she tried to hug it. The raccoon bit two of her fingers. The woman told the doctor that she left her canine impressions on the raccoon before it scampered away. After leaving the emergency department, the woman disappeared too. Although the raccoon's food-seeking behavior was normal, raccoon bites are taken very seriously and tracked to ensure completion of the vaccine series. Sally enlisted the help of PHN Paula because of her knack for finding people who don't want to be found. Through the woman's previous address, housing records, and relatives she was eventually found and completed PEP, but not before some anxious moments as it took several days to track her down.

Sally had the results of the third raccoon before the next conference call. It only served to increase her sense of urgency, a feeling that wouldn't leave until the control plan was underway. She read her list of agenda items to the participants of the second conference call:

1. Where should raccoons be trapped? Just in Central Park or in nearby parks as well?
2. Since the population of raccoons in Central Park was unknown, how many raccoons should be culled? Should they pick a number or a time period?
3. Who will perform the trapping, euthanasia, decapitation, and transportation?
4. How much will it cost and who will pay for it?
5. What will be the public message and who will deliver it?

Martin Lowney of the USDA and Bob Rudd, head of the NY Wadsworth Center Rabies Laboratory had joined the task force. They recommended using a one-mile radius around a central point defined by the locations of the first three raccoons as the trapping zone. This brought them well outside of the boundaries of Central Park. The group decided it was better to stay within the confines of the park, or parks if deemed necessary. The USDA offered up experienced local staff to handle the trapping. They could set fifty traps per night and suggested ten to fourteen nights might be enough depending on weather conditions and the raccoon population.

Sally nudged the group to the most difficult part of the plan. Once captured, the raccoons would need to be humanely euthanized, decapitated so their brains could be tested for the presence of rabies virus, and transported to the lab. ACC couldn't handle the volume in question. But both NYC and NY labs could test fifty raccoons per week. That necessitated a refrigeration plan to store specimens awaiting testing or a limit to only a portion of trapped raccoons, but someone still needed to perform the euthanasia and decapitation. The USDA stepped up again. Lowney would have to check with supervisors, but they could likely do the dirty work but would need a secure location to park their trailer, preferably within Central Park. NYC Parks was tasked with providing a secluded open-air workspace with a source of water.

These were not easy discussions. The Parks Department and their nonprofit partner, the CPC, were both anxious about rabies in the park but torn by the prospect of killing and disposing of hundreds of raccoons. That was bound to arouse public protest. Many of their donors and supporters were animal welfare activists or at least sympathetic to the cause. It was a financial risk they weren't willing to take. The trailer couldn't be parked on Central Park property. The task force then had to look for another place, but every agency they approached refused. Like a nuclear waste storage depot, no one wanted it in their backyard.

And the cost? No one seemed to know. The USDA thought their trapping staff time would come to around $5,000, maybe twice that including the staff needed to process the raccoons but that didn't include lab supplies, transportation, disposal, or a refrigeration truck. The line was silent when it came to footing the bill. No one said it but it likely wasn't far from their minds that epizootic raccoon rabies in Central Park was literally a black eye for NYC, on the scale of bed bugs in luxury hotels. The task force needed someone from the Mayor's Office with the fiscal and political clout to make this happen. Not only was Sally going to have to pitch the plan to the health commissioner and have him petition the mayor, but she was also nominated as spokesperson to handle media calls. A week had passed and there were still many crucial issues to be resolved, but a plan had been formulated.

By mid-December four more rabid raccoons turned up bringing the total to seven. One was found dead by the Harlem Meer, close to the location of the first rabid raccoon in August. Another was noted wandering on a softball field just north of the Great Lawn. It had suffered an abdominal wound and was in the last throes when the Conservancy worker hauled it off to be tested. The third was not far away from the second but on the east side and the fourth was found alive, but unresponsive, in nearby Morningside Park. The outbreak was expanding.

The task force convened three times in December and then not again until January 2010. The control plan still lacked a place to euthanize and prepare the raccoons for testing. City agencies with sufficient space close to Central Park, and even those far from the park, all declined to participate. Health Commissioner Farley was informed of the plan and the latest rabid raccoon count. He asked to speak with Richard Rosatte, who orchestrated a similar initiative in Ontario, the USDA, and the CDC. Commissioner Farley didn't think a yearly depopulation like what was done in Ontario could be sustained. Chuck Rupprecht of the CDC related a similar situation in Fairmount Park, Philadelphia, back in 1990. They used only TVR, no culling, and raccoon rabies was now controlled. Sally asked for the numbers, but none were published. However, the Philadelphia Department of Health reported only six rabid raccoons in the entire city between 2000–2008. While this experience was encouraging, Sally knew the Philadelphia outbreak was small and surveillance less aggressive. Would it be enough? The stakes were high. Failure and there would be enzootic rabies in Central Park. Just saying the words sent a shiver down her spine. Commissioner Farley asked why not conduct TVR with or without ORV. He asked the task force to consider a no-depopulation option.

Meanwhile, word of the plan leaked to the Humane Society, and the local field director of the Urban Wildlife Program contacted Sally. Boasting over 200,000 local members, she echoed some of the same concerns already known to the task force and added a claim not substantiated in the literature—nearly one-fifth of raccoons develop protective immunity to rabies infection. She asserted that culling would reduce the population of immune raccoons and worsen the situation. She also doubted the results of the Canadian experience. With the raccoon out of the bag, Sally had yet another concern on her mind.

Sally discussed the TVR-only plan with members of the task-force, and no one objected. Perhaps they were in a jolly mood since it was close to Christmas. More likely it came as a relief as no one enjoyed the prospect of executing hundreds of raccoons. They now had an enforceable plan but still needed to work out the details of contracts and find the money. By the end of 2009, there were eleven rabid raccoons in Central Park and nearby Morningside and Riverside Parks. No humans or pets had yet encountered a rabid raccoon. But that was about to change.

Near dusk on January 12, 2010, a middle-aged psychologist headed to his downtown office. His route took him through Central Park along the north shore of the Harlem Meer. As he exited onto Frawley Circle at Fifth Avenue, he heard what he at first took to be the growl of a dog. Looking up across the street he saw in the shadow of the Duke Ellington statue a raccoon. It was several yards away, still growling and staring at him. Then it charged. The psychologist instinctively swung his foot to kick the animal aside, but the raccoon latched onto his shoe. It is not unusual to hear stories of rabid animals with extraordinary strength, misguided determination, and a lack of sense for their own well-being. While attempting to shake loose the raccoon, the psychologist lost his balance and fell. As he reached for a fistful of fur, the raccoon bit his gloved thumb before he could manage to toss the raccoon discus-style into the park. The raccoon rolled to its feet and continued to stare him down before finally lumbering away. After he made it to the subway car, the man removed the glove and noticed blood. He had to visit two hospitals but received PEP and didn't contract rabies.

One week later, a man took his dog out for a walk in Central Park in the early evening hours. They were on the east side, walking the bridal path just a few yards from the Jacqueline Kennedy Onassis Reservoir, a location popular with runners and tourists. The dog was off the leash as Central Park rules permit dogs to roam off their leashes before 9:00 a.m. and after 9:00 p.m. A raccoon dashed out of the bushes and attacked the dog. The dog fought back, and the raccoon retreated. The dog suffered bites and scratches but fortunately had received rabies vaccination. Treatment required a booster dose and a precautionary forty-five-day home quarantine against a breakthrough infection.

It was early February and Sally was reviewing animal bite reports when she came across one that had been closed as not needing follow-up. She noticed a code indicating an exposure, so Sally asked staff to contact the woman. The sixty-one-year-old woman was an animal lover and had come across an ill raccoon in Central Park near Seventy-Ninth Street. It looked dehydrated so she tried to give it water by putting her wet finger in its mouth— yes, this really is what she did. She then brought the raccoon to ACC where it subsequently died. Testing was quickly arranged, and the raccoon tested positive. It would become the only raccoon versus dog or human encounter in which the animal was available for testing. The woman received PEP along with a request to alert the Parks Department or a licensed animal rehabber should she encounter a sick raccoon.

The NYC contract system is a myriad of checks and balances to ensure that the award process is fair, bids are competitively low, and city officials refrain from rewarding relatives, friends, or former employees. The oversight, while necessary, is glacially slow, six months wasn't unusual, and one must negotiate paperwork bottlenecks, fiscal auditing, legal review, and even background checks. Sally was warned that the USDA contract would take six months to work its way through the system. Unfortunately, there just isn't a good way to prioritize urgent contracts. But the situation couldn't wait. In six months, the next candidate for City Council from the Upper West Side might be a rabid raccoon.

TVR began on February 16, 2010, and concluded on April 9, 2010. Trap sites were selected based on reports of raccoon sightings or foraging for food in trash bins, evidence of dens, or scat. USDA trappers baited specially constructed cages with marshmallows. It turns out raccoons share more with humans than a predilection for urban living. They also have a sweet tooth. At the beginning of the TVR, approximately twenty traps were set in anticipation that the percentage of captured animals would be high. This increased to nearly sixty as the TVR program progressed. Upon entering the trap, the animal steps on a pressure-sensitive plate that triggers the door to snap close.

At sun-up each day a team of two or three USDA trappers made the rounds. First, they checked to see if the trap was occupied. If so, a check of the animal's health status came next. Raccoons are quite acclimated to humans and while in the trap they viewed their captors with calm curiosity, much like a toddler might view their parents from the confines of their playpen. The telltale signs of a rabid animal include drooling, unsteadiness of movement, trouble breathing, aggressiveness, and excessive licking which is a sign of dehydration. The trappers looked for ear tags of previously captured raccoons and checked for wounds incurred in a fight with a potentially rabid animal. On several occasions, trapped raccoons were already dead, having succumbed to rabies or another ailment.

Healthy raccoons were ear-tagged and vaccinated using a fork-like tool that pins them at one end of the cage allowing the worker to safely handle them. The trap was then pointed away from the workers and the door was released. Sick or injured raccoons were euthanized and sent for rabies testing. If a trap was found empty, it was checked to ensure it was operating correctly and then the bait was freshened if necessary. The TVR program operated for a total of 1,697 trap nights in Central, Morningside, and Riverside Parks. The days were long, often from sun to sundown.

In the early morning hours, as the TVR program was just getting underway, Sally was in the north end of Central Park by the Lasker Rink with two USDA staff. They were checking cages and getting captured raccoons ready for vaccination when she heard a woman scream. It was the kind of scream one might hear in a horror film and her first thought was that a rabid raccoon was attacking either the woman or her dog. The three took off in the direction of the scream and came upon a Malamute clutch-ing a raccoon in its jaws and shaking it mercilessly. The raccoon appeared unwell and when the owner got control over her dog, the raccoon wobbled away toward a creek and hid in a crevice between the rocks. The Malamute had been off its leash when it attacked the raccoon. The owner knew of the rabid raccoon prob-lem in the park but thought they were safe since raccoons are nocturnal. The USDA workers found the raccoon and it tested positive for rabies. The dog was given a booster shot and placed in home quarantine for forty-five days.

The number of raccoon-human encounters increased. In the last week of March 2010, a nineteen-year-old who just moved to the United States was visiting Central Park. He had never seen a raccoon and when one strolled by, he tried to pet it and got bitten. A little more than a week later a food cart vendor described a raccoon appearing out of nowhere; it ran at him and bit him on the shin. The raccoon then disappeared back into the woods. The final human encounter with a raccoon in Central Park occurred in June and was very much like the previous. A woman was sitting on a park bench near the east side entrance at Seventy-Second Street when a raccoon approached. She had no food, but the raccoon ran up and bit her on the ankle then took off for a nearby tree. The encounters kept us busy as we had to ensure that all affected persons completed the PEP regimen.

Of the 458 raccoons captured during TVR, 237 appeared well and were vaccinated, and 165 were recaptured one or more times. Before TVR began, from December 1, 2009, through February 15, 2010, approximately two rabid raccoons were found every three days. During the TVR program this increased to a little more than one per day and in the month following TVR that number dropped to less than one rabid raccoon every two days. In the last six months of 2010, there were five rabid raccoons found in Central Park compared to 135 during the first six months.

A second round of TVR aimed to inoculate the kits born in the spring as they became mobile. The program began in mid-September and finished in early November. It ended early because no unvaccinated raccoons were being trapped, a sign that good vaccination coverage had been achieved. During the second round, another 167 raccoons were inoculated bringing the total to 404. The new estimate of the Central Park raccoon population, based on the recapture rate of previously vaccinated raccoons during the second TVR, was 483. If accurate, it meant that 84% of the raccoon population had been vaccinated, higher than the estimated 65% needed to interrupt transmission. Although it is still too early to claim long-term success, the data suggests that the program had worked.

The TVR program's success in halting the spread of raccoon rabies in Central Park likely has more to do with the ecology of the park than with human ingenuity. Surrounded by tens of square miles of concrete and steel, Central Park is an isolated eco-system. Immigration of raccoons into the area is likely uncommon. Therefore, should a rabid raccoon find its way into the park the probability of encountering a susceptible raccoon would be low. This is the concept of herd immunity, the population protecting the health of the individual. It is how we control diseases such as measles and have eradicated smallpox from the planet. Raccoons in the wild usually live about two years. Because of the abundance of food and relative safety of Central Park, a raccoon's life span may be doubled.

Another round of TVR was repeated in the fall of 2011 when the next generation of raccoon kits began to explore their urban paradise. To ensure that rabies does not make a return to the park, the next phase of the raccoon rabies control plan consists of the use of ORV to cover areas of the park unsuitable for trapping. All involved, from park rangers to Sally to the owners of the esti-mated 1.5 million dogs in NYC, will need to remain vigilant.

The focus of this investigation was a response—halt the spread of raccoon rabies in Central Park. Other than hearing updates from Sally at the weekly outbreak meeting or asking questions when I'd pass her in the hallway, my role was merely as a fasci-nated spectator. The question of how the first rabid raccoon got to

Central Park troubled me. How could we prevent a return? Are we committed to an annual TVR program? There are a few theories of how raccoon rabies was introduced into Central Park. As occurred in Florida and the entire East Coast, the natural movement of raccoons has been quite efficient in spreading the virus. The three closest zones of enzootic raccoon rabies to Central Park are the boroughs of the Bronx, Queens, and Staten Island, and all are separated from the park by miles of concrete, steel, automobile traffic, and water. New York City truly is a city that doesn't sleep. A raccoon cruising across Madison Avenue would be noticed if not panic-stricken by taxicabs and buses.

The Bronx is the closest borough to Manhattan. The rabid raccoon found near 207th Street in August 2009, a mere eighteen blocks from the Bronx, lends support to this theory. Although the bridge distances—there are over a dozen bridges connecting the Bronx to Manhattan—are short, the terrain is not ideal raccoon habitat. There is not much in the way of trees or cover. However, there is a Metro-North train tunnel that passes from the Bronx into Manhattan and courses through Riverside Park. But traps set along this corridor did not capture any raccoons. If the initial rabid raccoon entered Manhattan from the Bronx and then into Riverside Park, we would expect that the height of the epizootic would be in Riverside and not in Central Park. The second theory is that an illegal translocation occurred. This means that a captured raccoon from the Bronx, Queens, or Staten Island, or somewhere else, was driven into Central Park and released. There are parks in the Bronx, Queens, and Staten Island, so it seems unlikely that a person would drive into the insane traffic of Manhattan and risk being spotted breaking the law. However, former presidential candidate Robert F. Kennedy, Jr. recently admitted to dumping a deceased bear cub in Central Park in 2014, so it is not beyond the realm of possibility.[65]

After softball games, I'd often sit in Central Park until well after sundown. It was partly the defiant kid in me refusing to admit playtime was over and partly to savor the precious moments of summer in the city. I've had my share of sports injuries and didn't know how much longer I'd be able to enjoy softball in the park. In the fading and angled evening light the colors become brilliant. The departure of the crowds brings a rare peace to the Great Lawn. On my way out of the park, I'd invariably pass trucks loading up the food carts. I wondered, where did the carts go to spend the night?

The third theory of how raccoon rabies was introduced to Central Park is an accidental translocation. Raccoons have been known to stow away on trucks and show up at garbage dumps. During the warm weather months, trucks enter Central Park daily from the other boroughs to drop off mobile food vendor carts and bring in supplies. We inquired, and no one reported seeing a raccoon stowaway. There is, however, no monitoring system.

The issue remains that something unusual must have occurred in NYC in 2009. Raccoon rabies arrived in the city via Staten Island in March of 1992. For the previous seventeen years, it had not found its way into Central Park. Why now? Only time will tell if it takes annual TVR programs to control raccoon rabies, or if it has been successfully eradicated.

Rabid animals, including raccoons, continue to show up throughout NYC. Between four and thirty positive raccoons per year have been found from 2014–2023. mostly in the Bronx and Staten Island. In 2013, rabid raccoons were found in Inwood and Fort Tryon Parks in the very northern tip of Manhattan. The health department responded with TVR followed by annual rounds of ORV, and I joined the team for a walk in the park tossing the smelly bait-ORV packs into the woods. The good news is that there hasn't been a rabies positive raccoon found in Central Park since 2011.

CHAPTER 10

Dying to Be Beautiful

Beauty is big business. Worldwide revenue for non-surgical interventions is estimated to be $65 billion.[66] Plastic surgery revenue alone in the United States is valued at $25 billion.[67] Celebrities and actors have reportedly spent thousands of dollars on cosmetic procedures.[68,69] It's lucrative but to cash in you must have a state-issued license to practice medicine. Obtaining a medical license requires completing four years of medical school, passing a series of three US medical licensing examinations, and fulfilling at least one year of hospital residency. To become board-certified in plastic surgery, you must do six or more years of training plus a certification exam. It's a long, expensive, and arduous process that is even more difficult for foreign medical school graduates.

Where there is demand, the black market will fill the void. Most beauty services are for aesthetics, and people seek low-cost enhancements such as a fuller bosom, slimmer waist, more shapely thighs and buttocks. The shadowy medical procedures are conducted in apartments, hotel rooms, and even within legitimate businesses. The equipment used isn't standard medical quality and sanitary precautions are absent. The costs are from a few hundreds to thousands of dollars, far cheaper than licensed care in bona fide medical facilities. The results can be catastrophic.

In 2002, a cluster of *Mycobacterium abscessus* infections were detected in NYC among Latinx women who all underwent cosmetic injections. *M. abscessus* is a soil-dwelling organism related to tuberculosis and the Bureau of Tuberculosis Control, with assistance from the CDC, conducted the investigation. A total of twenty-five persons were affected with body parts including the face, arms, breasts, hips, abdomen, hips, and buttocks. The chemicals injected were traced to Venezuela. Two assailants were arrested and identified as a Venezuelan couple who did not possess licenses to practice medicine in the United States.[70] The couple operated out of an East Side Manhattan apartment and flew back and forth to Venezuela to smuggle non-FDA-approved medications into the country. They pleaded guilty to first-degree reckless endangerment and were sentenced to two to seven years in prison, followed by deportation.

The DODs first investigated illegal medical practice in January of 2006. Pam Kellner, RN, MPH took the lead. Pam's ancestors were from Scotland and arrived in America via Canada in the 1600s. She grew up on a small farm in the Berkshires of Western Massachusetts and had an interest in nursing from a young age when she volunteered as a candy striper in the local hospital. Pam moved to NYC, attended nursing school, modeled by day and nursed at night before returning to school to obtain a master's degree in public health from Columbia University. She joined the department in 1992 to help combat the tuberculosis epidemic and transferred to the DODs in 2003. We had received a report of *Mycobacterium fortuitum*, which like *M. abscessus*, is a soil-dwelling mycobacterium related to tuberculosis. The woman had undergone several mesotherapy procedures at Maria Vasco

Aesthetics, a Queens beauty salon. Mesotherapy involves the injection of chemicals into the skin ostensibly to dissolve fat. A dubious procedure at best. When Pam arrived at the second-floor office in Jackson Heights, Queens, with NYPD, she found a busy hair salon. The staff and patrons were stunned to see her accompanied by uniformed officers. In one corner of the salon was a walled-off office approximately 10 x 6. Barricaded inside was Marcia Cabrera, a NY-licensed cosmetologist and proprietor of the alleged illegal medical practice. Ms. Cabrera's lawyer appeared and after the NYPD assured him that they were not there to arrest Ms. Cabrera, Pam gained access to the office. Among the medical supplies she found were vials of silicone oil, many of which were punctured with a needle and left open and exposed to air and stored haphazardly in the refrigerator. Ms. Cabrera was alleged to be administering injections, prescribing antibiotics, and performing other procedures that required medical training and licensure. Needles were found disposed of in the regular trash, a violation of medical waste regulations. Materials were confiscated and Ms. Cabrera was issued a health commissioner order to cease operations. The complainant did not wish to pursue charges so there was no criminal prosecution.

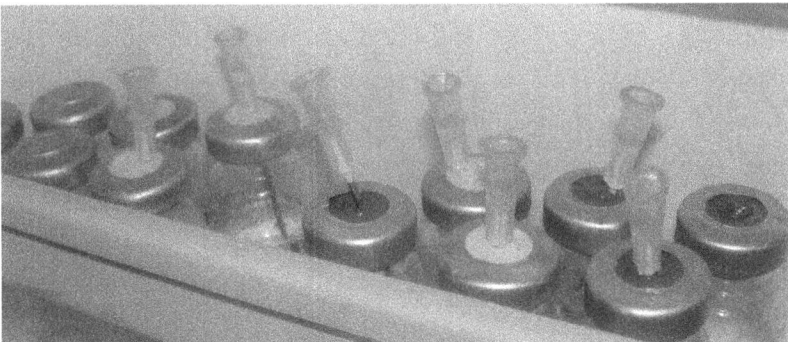

Freezer shelf with silicone vials not properly stored. Images from Maria Vasco Aesthetics.

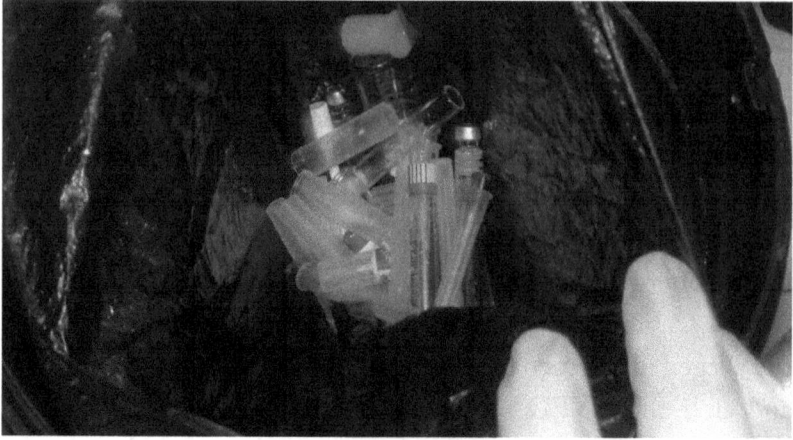

Trash can with medical waste. Images from Maria Vasco Aesthetics.

The most extensive illegal medical practice investigation occurred in 2010. Dr. Lew Soloff was serving as the BCD doctor-of-the-week; a rotation of medical epidemiologists who triaged and responded to calls from providers, city officials, and the public. He took the initial call on a late March afternoon. The caller was a surgical resident from a Queens hospital and told Lew about a twenty-three-year-old woman who had been admitted with bilateral buttock abscesses. A week before she presented to the hospital the woman had undergone liposuction. Fat was removed from her belly and then reinserted into her buttocks to create a fuller appearance. Lew learned that the woman had pain and a fever of 103°F and required surgical drainage of the abscesses which were quite large—about the size of a pack of cigarettes each. Lew, who in addition to his job with the D❂Ds, also worked as an emergency department physician, visited the hospital to review the medical record and interview the patient.

The patient told Lew that on the advice of a friend, she went to Bel Stetika, a spa located in the Corona Section of Queens. The procedure was performed by the owner, Barbara Nieto, and involved the use of local anesthesia, incisions in her abdomen to remove fat, and then incisions in her buttocks to reinsert the removed fat. It was done in an ordinary room, and she was able to leave fifteen minutes after completion. She paid $500 in cash. The patient returned to Bel Stetika each day for the next three days due to pain and received massage on the surgical sites. After the third visit, she was advised to go to the emergency department but was told not to mention the procedure.

Non-licensed medical practice isn't covered under the NY Office of Professional Medical Conduct (OPMC) who have oversight responsibility of physicians. Unless the act causes an infection that a healthcare provider chooses to report, we won't hear about it. Technically, the act is considered a crime and is in the jurisdiction of the police. However, the police don't possess the necessary medical expertise or resources to investigate every complaint or employ prevention tactics. As a result, illegal medical practice operates largely with impunity.

Lew's primary job with the D☉Ds was helping hospitals prepare for natural and intentional disasters, so he turned the investigation over to me. I enlisted the assistance of Jennifer Baumgartner, a data scientist who had been serving as the research scientist-of-the-week. Jen joined the department in 2004 and previously worked for the STI and Information Technology Bureaus before joining BCD's hepatitis unit. She received her MSPH from the University of Utah and worked briefly as a laboratory technician in Salt Lake City before coming to NYC. Her laboratory experience would prove quite useful as she oversaw the Electronic Clinical Laboratory Reporting System. Jen sat two rows over, and like mine, her cubicle faced the corridor which meant that staff routinely stopped by to chat. I guess that meant she never had to leave her seat to be social because that's where one could always find her, plugging away at her keyboard, eyes glued to the screen, searching for errors in SAS code and explanations for missing lab reports. Jen comes from a large family and generally only speaks when she has something to say, which never includes an unkind word. She was a member, as was I, of the D✪D curmudgeon club, which of course never met nor had any official members. We followed Groucho Marx's advice of never joining a club that would have us as a member.

HaeNa Waechter was also enlisted to help with the investigation. HaeNa was recently hired as an epidemiologist with BCD's foodborne unit after completing the Applied Epidemiology Fellowship with us. A native of Brooklyn, and a former high school softball player, HaeNa received her BA from Carnegie Mellon University and her MPH from Columbia University. HaeNa had played catcher, so she was adept at not letting things get past her. A useful skill as a D✪D. Getting to a softball field in NYC often takes perseverance, another trait that made HaeNa indispensable to the team. We reached out to NYPD and Detectives Failla and Neacy from the major case squad were assigned to the case.

While arranging with the NYPD and our legal department to visit the facility, we sought to locate others who may have been injured by this unlicensed practitioner. We found a civil complaint lodged by a Queens woman who received injections in 2009, but she declined to assist with our investigation. An anonymous complaint had been received by OPMC back in 2008, but because Barbara Nieto did not have a medical license, the complaint was not investigated.

The site visit, or raid as the NYPD called it, occurred on April 8, 2010. It was led by Jennifer and Dr. Bindy Crouch, a physician who worked in the hospital readiness unit of BCD with Lew.

Bindy's path to becoming a D✪D is a most fascinating one.

She was born in Vietnam in 1974 just as the war was ending, and South Vietnam was in crisis. Her parents, unable to care for her, delivered her to an orphanage. She was adopted by an American family through Operation Babylift. In April 1975, as Saigon was falling, the first Operation Babylift flight took off but crashed into a rice field killing most of the children and crew members. Years later, at a Babylift reunion, Bindy would learn that she was likely on that doomed flight and one of the few crash survivors. Bindy grew up in Massachusetts and has been back to Vietnam several times, once for a medical school elective, and again to provide medical care in an orphanage.

Detectives Failla and Neacy had a search warrant and Bindy had our equivalent, a Commissioner's Order. Several patients were in the waiting room and others were in treatment rooms. None were receiving treatments that would require a medical license, but all were asked if they needed medical services. None did. An inventory of supplies was made, and photographs were taken. Among the items found that suggested medical procedures were taking place were lidocaine vials used for local anesthesia when doing surgical procedures, Botox, mesotherapy drugs, needles, syringes, intravenous infusion solutions, and the antidepressant drug fluoxetine (brand name is Prozac). No liposuction equipment was found, however, a plastic tube with a connector was found that could be used for liposuction

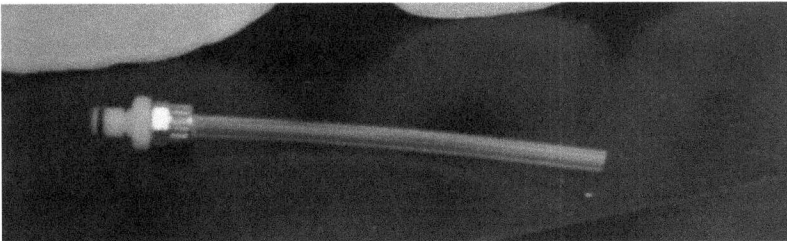

Plastic Tubing Confiscated from Bel Stetika Spa

As part of the investigation, Jen and HaeNa collected the appointment logs and designed a questionnaire to understand the procedures that were performed and what, if any harms, may have occurred. Over 400 clients were contacted and just under half consented to be interviewed. Over 95% were women and 60% had undergone one or more invasive procedures that required medical training and licensure, most commonly injection of fillers to alter body contour, mesotherapy, and liposuction. About a third of clients experienced adverse effects, such as pain, swelling, and redness. More serious side effects such as infections requiring medical treatment and scarring occurred in less than 10% of clients. Oral medications dispensed from Bell Stetika Spa ranged from antibiotics to intravenous infusions of vitamin cocktails.

One patient, a child, received a facial injection of their own blood. The procedure was advertised on their website as PRP–Plasma Rica en Plaquetas for $300. Platelet-rich plasma (PRP) is a procedure in which a patient's blood is removed and centrifuged to separate out cells and concentrate platelets and plasma which is then injected, typically into joints, to relieve pain or regenerate tissues. It must be done with strict adherence to sterile technique. In 2010, it was an emerging therapy requiring a level of expertise that most physicians, let alone unlicensed individuals, didn't possess. The presence of a centrifuge in the spa supports that this was the procedure that was provided. Based on our investigation, New York State suspended Barbara Nieto's business license and set a date for a hearing to decide whether it should be revoked.

Detective Failla called me in the early evening of Friday, April 9, 2010, while I was at the gym. They had located a second site run by Ms. Nieto, Perfect Image Aesthetics on Junction Boulevard in Queens. They asked that I meet them there, so I headed back to my apartment to shower, but by the time I was ready to head out,

Detective Failla called me back. The accused had rented a room at the location, but no equipment was found.

It took two years for the case to work its way through the legal system. Bindy testified before the Queens County Grand Jury in March 2011 which returned an indictment on the following charges:

PL 120.05-4 ASSAULT IN THE SECOND DEGREE
PL 120.05-6 ASSAULT IN THE SECOND DEGREE
PL 120.25 RECKLESS ENDANGERMENT IN THE
  FIRST DEGREE
ED LAW 6512-1 UNAUTHORIZED PRACTICE A
  CRIME

A year later, I was informed as supervisor of the investigation that my testimony was needed, and Queens Assistant District Attorney (ADA) Allison Wright prepared me for trial. I had been a public health witness before in St. Louis. That case dealt with a delinquent landlord whose neglect of his properties resulted in the lead poisoning of children. ADA Wright explained that my testimony would proceed similarly to what is depicted in TV legal shows. First, I would describe my job at the department and my training, where I went to medical school and did residency, as well as any other pertinent training, such as master's degree coursework and the Epidemiology in Action Course I took at the CDC. ADA Wright would further ask about my work experience, and my current duties, specifically as they pertained to illegal medical practice. Once my public health credentials were entered into the record, she'd request that I be qualified as an expert witness. The defense attorney would have the opportunity to ask me questions or even object to my qualification as an expert, but this would likely not be sustained by the judge. Then ADA Wright would ask me to describe the events: How did we come to learn about the illegal practice of medicine? What steps did we take to investigate? What did we find? What evidence was collected? I'd review the photos Jennifer took and explain the nature of the procedures we believed the defendant had been doing that required medical licensure.

The trial was set to begin on April 25, 2012, but the defense attorney was representing a homicide defendant and requested a postponement. The extra time was fortuitous as the district attorney and defendant worked out a plea agreement and avoided a trial. In the plea agreement, announced in a press release on May 30, 2012, Ms. Nieto admitted to:

> *Taking the patient into a room with a machine connected with several hoses. Ms. Nieto injected the woman with a substance that was supposed to help with pain, then cut an opening in her stomach area, and used the machine to suction fat from her stomach area. Nieto then injected the woman in the buttocks with a supposed pain-relieving substance and then, making two incisions, reinserted the fat into her buttocks. Ms. Nieto completed the medical procedures by stitching up the holes in the woman's stomach area and buttocks.* [71]

In the plea agreement announced in the Queens District Attorney's press release Ms. Nieto pled guilty to unlawful medical practice and assault and would spend two years in jail followed by three years of post-release supervision. She was ordered to pay $180,000 in fines and restitution to her clients. [72]

Unfortunately, this was not the last time an illegal medical practice injured someone in NYC. Whalesca Castillo was alleged to have practiced medicine illegally in the Bronx for years.[73] In 2012, she spent nine months in federal prison, but upon her release, she resumed impersonating a medical professional. She was caught again in 2018 but this time with deadly consequences. She injected silicone oil into forty-eight-year-old Lesbia Ayala who then suffered an embolism and died.[74] Ms. Castillo was sentenced to four to eight years in prison.[75]

In April 2009, a twenty-eight-year-old transgender NYC woman paid an unlicensed medical practitioner to inject 500 ml of a mixture of silicone and castor bean oil into her thighs and buttocks. Within hours she had a headache and chest and abdominal pain. Twelve hours later she was urinating blood, and her skin turned yellow, requiring hospitalization for liver and kidney failure. The woman survived but required dialysis until her kidney function returned to normal.[76]

A rap artist using the moniker the Black Madam injected industrial-grade silicone oil into the buttocks of Claudia Aderotimi, a British dancer, in a hotel room near the Philadelphia airport in 2011. Twelve hours later the woman developed difficulty breathing. The silicone oil had migrated into her bloodstream and lodged in her lungs causing a pulmonary embolism which precipitated cardiac arrest. Ms. Aderotimi died. She was twenty years old. The perpetrator went into hiding but soon resumed her practice. She was eventually caught, tried, found guilty of third-degree murder, and sentenced to ten to twenty years in prison.[77, 78]

Deaths due to illegal medical practice have occurred in New York, Texas, Florida, and California. While deaths get the headlines, many victims, mostly women, suffer years of pain, disfigurement, and kidney and lung problems. Many don't report the injuries to authorities out of fear, embarrassment, or an unwillingness to cause trouble. Using an unlicensed medical practitioner for cosmetic enhancement may save money, but the risks are far too great to sacrifice one's health and well-being.

CHAPTER 11

The Mummy of Queens

It began with the clank of metal on metal. The construction workers thought the backhoe's bucket had struck an old pipe. And then feet slid into view. They were working in an abandoned lot in Elmhurst, Queens, late on the afternoon of October 4, 2011. The condition of the remains suggested a recent death and since organized crime was known to dispose of people in construction sites, allegedly under cement, the supervisor notified the police who called the OCME. It was dark by the time detectives and paramedics arrived. But it soon became obvious that these were no ordinary human remains.

The OCME informed Scott Warnasch, their forensic anthropologist. When he arrived on the scene, he quickly determined that the metal wasn't a pipe, but an iron coffin. It dated back to the mid-nineteenth century. Iron coffins were in favor in the 1850s, before embalming technology, and were used by the wealthy to preserve bodies when transported over great distances, and in cases of suspected communicable diseases. Iron coffins were constructed to be airtight, preventing organisms from the surrounding soil to hasten decomposition.

The lot at 90-15 Corona Avenue had been the location of St.

Mark's African Methodist Episcopal (AME) Church and cemetery. The well-preserved remains appeared to be those of a young African American woman. Inspection of her skin provided a clue to her cause of death. There were numerous raised bumps, some of which had dimpled centers: characteristic of smallpox. The body was removed and transported to the Queens Medical Examiner's Office. The CDC and DODs were called.

Smallpox had been a disease only of humans, with no environmental or animal reservoir. *Had been* because it no longer exists in nature. A worldwide vaccine campaign was undertaken and achieved the unthinkable: complete eradication. The last naturally occurring case of smallpox occurred in 1977 in Somalia. Nevertheless, scientists continued to study the virus throughout the last century and stocks are believed to remain in laboratories in Russia and the United States. Some concern exists that the deadly scourge could make a return, perhaps from well-preserved human remains. An English physician claimed that during the demolition of a smallpox hospital prior to the eradication, a worker, having no other plausible explanation, contracted the disease.[79] In yet another bizarre tale reported in the English medical literature, multiple attendees of a 1759 funeral contracted smallpox when a thirty-year-old coffin of a smallpox victim was accidentally entered by a spade.[80] In Ohio in the 1860s, a grave robber named Old Cunny deliberately provided a smallpox corpse to a medical school to exact revenge on mischievous medical students. Several students reportedly subsequently contracted the disease.[81]

Smallpox is caused by the virus *Variola major.* Seven to seventeen days after exposure, the prodrome begins with a fever as high as 105°F and is accompanied by severe muscle aches, headache, anorexia, and prostration. After a few days, the rash begins, first as flat red spots but progresses from papules to vesicles to pustules over two weeks. Smallpox is transmitted primarily in two ways: via respiratory droplets to individuals in close and prolonged proximity, and by contact with the rash. A person becomes infective once the rash appears in the throat (enanthem) and is most infectious during the first week of illness. Death occurs in about one-third of those infected.

The prevention of smallpox dates to ancient civilizations. It was known that the healed scabs from survivors could be used to inoculate others. The process is called variolation and was intended to inflict a milder version of the illness and provoke a lifelong protective immune response. Variolation was not entirely safe as some recipients contracted smallpox and developed complications or died. At the end of the seventeenth century, Edward Jenner, an English physician, noted that while milkmaids had facial complexions unblemished by smallpox scars, their hands were not so spared. He discovered cowpox, a virus related to smallpox, that is non fatal to humans. He collected specimens from newly infected milkmaids and developed a new procedure to prevent smallpox. He named its vaccination after *vacca*, the Latin word for cow. Vaccination was slow to achieve acceptance but by the 1850s it was widely practiced in New York while variolation had been banned by an 1816 state law.

Smallpox has likely killed more humans than any other infectious disease, however, since tuberculosis and malaria still exist, they may eventually eclipse its deadly tally. Years after vaccine campaigns eliminated smallpox from the world, health officials petitioned governments holding the virus to destroy all stocks. While most nations complied, the virus remains frozen in research labs in the United States and Russia. In the past several decades, there has been interest in investigating the long-term viability of smallpox. Perhaps this interest was stimulated by research done in the Netherlands in the 1950s. The researchers collected scabs from persons sickened during an outbreak of *Variola minor*, smallpox's less severe relative. They stored the scabs in a lab at room temperature and tested the virus's viability for several years. The virus remained viable for thirteen years and perhaps would have survived longer had they not run out of scabs and terminated the study.[82]

In May of 2011, a museum in Virginia, while sorting through holdings to create an exhibit, came across an envelope from 1876. Inside was a letter and a scab. The letter stated that the scab could be used to vaccinate twelve individuals. It turned out to be a vaccination scab and harmless.[83] Mid-sixteenth century remains from Naples, Italy; a Peruvian mummy from 950; and even Ramses V have all been tested, and while some identified putative viral particles, none found a viable virus.[84] But what if the scabs had been preserved frozen? Similar to how smallpox is stored in research labs? Could it be thawed and cause an outbreak? In 2004, an archaeological dig in Siberian permafrost uncovered a mass grave. Smallpox DNA fragments were recovered, but again the virus was not viable.[85]

The CDC decided to travel to NYC and test the mummy for smallpox. I was assigned to observe the autopsy of the 160-year-old woman and take photographs. I drew the assignment because back in 2003, at the height of bioterrorism concerns, I volunteered to be re-vaccinated for smallpox. There had been a push to get first responders and healthcare workers vaccinated because the invasion of Iraq had stirred fears of bioterrorism.

Before entering the autopsy suite, we all donned special suits provided by the CDC. Hoods covered our heads and booties our feet. We also wore double gloves, high-efficiency masks, and face shields. The CDC laid out on the stainless-steel table a row of sampling vials. The odor was like nothing I had ever encountered—an acrid mix of ammonia and metal. Pathologist Dr. Corinne Ambrosi, from the Queens Medical Examiner's office, orchestrated the procedure. The woman's clothing was remarkably intact—a white gown, chemise, cap, and knee-high socks. Her hair was held in place by a comb. All of these were preserved for archaeological analysis.

The skin was a dark, reddish brown, perhaps from having absorbed rust from the iron coffin. It had the texture of leather. Her hair and features suggested African American heritage. Upon closer inspection, we saw raised, round papules approximately one-eighth inch in diameter. The centers of the dimples were darkened and umbilicated. There were hundreds of papules on her scalp and extremities. Upon internal exam, no organs remained. Tissue samples were obtained including hair and a tooth. The tests failed to find any remnant of smallpox. Neither smallpox nor human DNA was recovered, all had degraded.

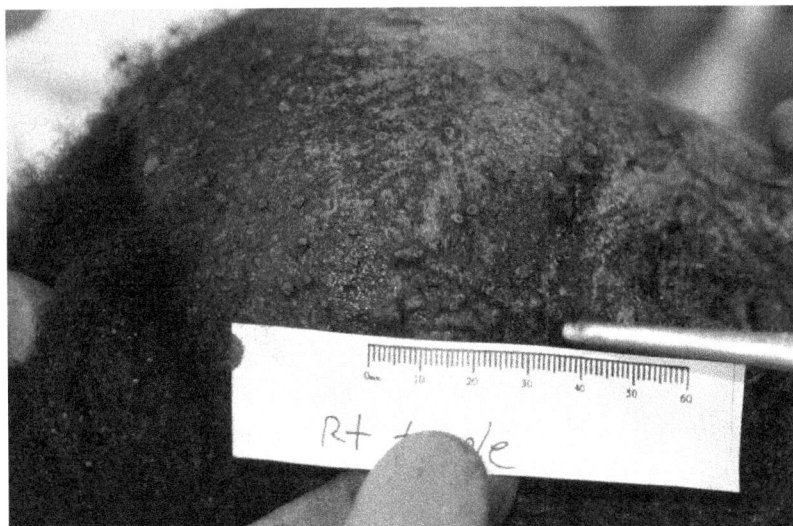

Examination of the scalp of the woman found in iron coffin showing smallpox rash

This was a much different type of D⊗D investigation. For starters, there was no one to interview. No medical records to review. No secondary cases to track backward to find the source. No one to isolate or quarantine. Had the testing identified a viable virus it would have triggered actions, but no interventions were needed. It also wasn't our case to investigate. The identity of the woman was unknown, there were no grave markings, and the iron coffin bore no identification plate.

The property at 90-15 Corona Avenue in Queens was within one of the earliest free, African American communities in the United States. In 1828, William and Jane Hunter deeded part of their Newtown family farm to the United African Society to erect a church. Alongside the church was a burial ground that in 1873 was part of the African Methodist Episcopal Church. In the early 1900s, the church's name changed to St. Mark's AME Church and was located at Corona Avenue west of Ninety-First Street. The church then moved in 1929 and applied for a city permit to relocate those interred in the cemetery, but the request was denied. Still, some remains were moved, but an estimated 300 burials are still present. In 1931, the cemetery disappeared from maps and those interred were forgotten. St. Mark's AME Church eventually moved to Jackson Heights and cemetery records were lost.

There were two questions remaining about the mummy. The woman's identity and how she contracted smallpox. Scott Warnasch pursued the first and I considered the latter. Warnasch arranged to have the woman examined using modern radiology. Her hair and tooth were sent to a geochemist. The exams estimated her age at the time of death based on her bone structures to be between twenty-five and thirty years old. She had mild osteo-arthritis which suggested that she had not been subjected to hard labor. Slavery had been abolished in New York in 1827 and the woman likely belonged to the free Black community in Newtown. The iron coffin was the best clue to her identity.

Warnasch had encountered iron coffins before, in fact, it had become his passion.[86] He was a consultant in 2005 when two iron coffins were unearthed in Newark, NJ, during construction for a hockey arena.[87] He suspected the manufacturer of the Queens iron coffin was Dunbar Fisk. Fisk had moved to NYC around 1840, invented an airtight stove, and built a stove manufacturing business. He bought land and built a home in Newtown, a hamlet in the county of Queens which was not yet part of NYC. He began making iron coffins after his brother's untimely death in the Deep South. Embalming hadn't been invented and bodies could not be transported great distances. The airtight iron coffin resolved the problem of rapid decomposition. The coffin lid was bolted in place and then sealed with molten lead. A glass window at the head allowed for viewing and it too would be covered and sealed before burial.

Warnasch's suspicions were confirmed when he located and examined the footplate of the coffin. It bore the Fisk patent stamp, plus another clue. The stamp was askew, a defect that probably meant it couldn't be sold. Iron caskets were expensive. A pine casket in 1850 cost around $2 whereas the iron version cost twenty to fifty times as much. Only the wealthy and famous were customers, Dolly Madison being the most noteworthy.

William M. Raymond was Dunbar's brother-in-law and lived next door in Newtown. Fisk and Dunbar both appear in the 1850 census as heads of households. Fisk was thirty-two years old, and his occupation was listed as a stove maker whereas Raymond was twenty-seven years old, and his occupation was listed as none. Fisk died months after the 1850 census from a chronic intestinal condition and likely pneumonia he contracted after saving a child from drowning in the East River. Sometime before his death, Dunbar took on Raymond as a business partner. When Warnasch viewed the Fisk and Raymond family members listed in the 1850 census he noticed that two African Americans lived in the Raymond household. One was a thirty-five-year-old male named Henry Peterson; the other was a twenty-six-year-old woman named Martha Peterson. Martha Peterson's age fits with the estimate of the woman found in the iron coffin and she did not again appear in the 1860 census suggesting she perhaps had died. So, who were Henry and Martha Peterson? Siblings, or husband and wife? Were they employed by the Raymonds?

To answer this Warnasch had to further go back in time. John and Jane Banker Peterson were residents of Newtown and prominent figures in the free African American community. Born in 1800 and 1798 respectively, they had several children. In the 1850 census, five children were listed in their household: daughters Mary (twenty-two years), Josephine (twenty years), and Harriet (sixteen years); and sons Elisha (eighteen years) and John (ten years).[88] Going back to previous census records, John Peterson and family appear in documents from 1830 and 1840, but for those censuses, the names and exact ages of African American children were not recorded. However, both recorded categories of children by age and sex. In 1830, five Peterson children were listed: two males between the ages of ten and twenty-three; one male under ten; and two females under ten years old.[89] In 1840, again five children were listed: two males under ten; one female between ten and twenty-three; and two females under ten years old. Martha would have been six years old in 1830 and could be one of the two girls listed under ten years old.[90] Mary might be the other, and perhaps the census was conducted prior to the birth of Josephine.

Henry would have been fifteen years old and could be one of the boys listed as between ten and twenty-three years old. Mortality for children in the nineteenth century was quite high, especially among African Americans. So, the second male between the ages of ten and twenty-three in the 1830 census might be a child who subsequently died. But since John would have been fifteen years old at the time of Henry's birth, it has been suggested that Henry might have been a child of Jane from a previous relationship.

Moving to the 1840 census, Martha would have been sixteen years old and might have found work outside of the Peterson home, therefore making her not present in the Peterson family census listing. However, Martha Peterson was not found in any other household. Mary, who would have been twelve, could be the one daughter listed in the ten to twenty-three range. Henry at twenty-five would most certainly have left the household.

The last piece of evidence suggesting that the woman in the iron coffin was Martha Peterson comes from the 1870 census. Elisha Peterson, who appears in the 1850 household of John Peterson, named one of his daughters Martha, perhaps in memory of his older sister.[91] Henry Peterson doesn't appear in the 1860 census. It is possible that he too died of smallpox or some other ailment.

How did Martha Peterson contract smallpox? While the disease was certainly present in NYC and surrounding counties, it was not an epidemic in the mid-eighteenth century. In 1850, there were 241 reported smallpox deaths in NYC, which translates to about 800 cases or 1.4 cases per 1,000 population (30% mortality rate; NYC population was 590,000). But in 1851 the number of deaths more than doubled to 586. By then, NYC was more densely populated than Queens so smallpox in Newtown, which had an estimated population of 2,000, was likely an uncommon event.

The mid-nineteenth century was also a time of great migration. It was not uncommon for smallpox to appear on ships resulting in quarantine and the vaccination of others. Ports were a notorious place for infectious disease to land. The city's government offered free vaccination to residents through its dispensaries, and efforts focused on the poor and immigrants. The same level of public service was not available in Queens, however, families with means could likely obtain vaccinations if they so desired. There was then, as now, a reticence by many to be vaccinated.

The last smallpox outbreak in NYC occurred in 1947. An American couple living in Mexico for several years boarded a bus in Mexico City for NYC. The bus made stops in Dallas, St. Louis, Cincinnati, and Pittsburgh. The husband took ill en route and developed a rash three days before arriving in NYC. He transmitted the disease to three patients during his hospitalization, and two of those patients transmitted smallpox to another eight persons—all were connected to healthcare. No one on the bus, in the hotel where the couple stayed, or persons who encountered them when they toured NYC, got ill. Oddly, the wife remained well. However, three people died, including the index case. The NYC Health Department in return vaccinated over 6 million people in the span of five weeks.[92]

As a household servant in the Raymond home, what activities would Martha have done to bring her into contact with a contagious case? Smallpox requires prolonged contact, like that of a family member or a caretaker. Caring for a smallpox case is a risk. The Raymond children were born in 1854, 1860, and 1864. Martha Peterson was believed to have died before 1854. If Martha's duties were as a domestic, which included cleaning, laundry, and perhaps cooking, how might she have encountered smallpox? A clue came from chemistry.

As part of the investigation, Warnasch provided samples to Dr. Rhonda Quinn for geochemical analysis. The tests of hair and teeth compared the presence of various elements and isotopes. The strontium concentration in her hair was near the maximum level found in people living today.[93] The findings are consistent with shellfish in the diet. Oysters happened to be a huge commodity in NYC in the 1850s. One of the most well-known oyster purveyors was Thomas Downing, a free African American who opened an oyster house on Broad Street in Lower Manhattan in 1819. By 1850, Downing's restaurant was renowned and catered to high-end clientele.

It seems unlikely that a servant from Queens would make the several-stage coach trip to Lower Manhattan for oysters when there were options closer to home. In the mid-nineteenth century, roads called turnpikes were being built in Queens. One of those roads connected Newtown with Flushing and another connected Newtown to Jamaica. Oysterman was a common occupation among free Blacks and both Flushing and Jamaica had bays with oyster beds. Whether Martha encountered smallpox while dining out or in travels to purchase supplies for the Raymond family will remain a matter of conjecture. The story of the woman in the iron coffin was featured in an episode of the PBS show, *Secrets of the Dead*.[94] Forensic imaging artist Joe Mullins's rendering of Martha Peterson can be found on numerous websites.[95]

CHAPTER 12

South Bronx in the Crosshairs Again

Late July in NYC can be sticky and uncomfortable. The maximum daily July temperature in the city during the first decade of the twenty-first century ranged between 87-97°F. However, between 2010–2014, the maximum temperature topped 100°F three times.[96] Coworkers questioned how I could bike to work in the heat and humidity, made worse by the cabs and cars. I'd tell them I preferred sweating in bike shorts and a Dri-Fit t-shirt to sweltering on subway platforms in work clothes. A bad day biking beats any day on the subway. Plus, we had a locker room with showers at our Long Island City headquarters where we moved in 2011. I'm an early riser and developed a routine. I'd prepare lunch and pack work clothes the night before. I'd leave my apartment at 6:30 a.m. before traffic became too treacherous, bike crosstown through Central Park, over the Queensboro Bridge, and shower to be at my desk before 8 a.m. I kept a towel at work and let it air dry in a hidden spot behind the waist-high file cabinets that lined the floor-to-ceiling windows by my cubicle. Early hours at the department are quiet and the best time to think. July was even quieter than usual because staff generally took their vacations in the summer. The work, however, didn't go on vacation.

The weather wasn't the only thing making us sticky and uncomfortable that summer. In the final weeks of July 2015, we were still triaging and monitoring sick travelers from West Africa for possible Ebola. The largest outbreak of Ebola was still raging in Guinea, Liberia, and Sierra Leone, and had seeded cases in seven countries, including the United States.[97] NYC had one imported case in a returning, volunteer healthcare worker in the fall of 2014. On average, we were receiving three to five each week from worried providers about patients suspected of having Ebola. Each call took several hours to process and evaluate if testing was needed. Test results took several days to return.

The second week of July was my turn to be the doctor-of-the-week. The Ebola Call Center referred a patient who had just returned from visiting Guinea. He had body aches and low-grade fever along with dark urine. He wanted to go to an emergency room in the Bronx. The man had been in Guinea for a month and hadn't taken malaria prophylaxis. He denied the risk factors of contact with anyone ill or a known case of Ebola and hadn't attended a funeral or consumed bush meat. He was also having chills. I notified the hospital, and they donned personal protective equipment to meet the patient in the ambulance bay so they could guide him through a side entrance to the isolation unit. A few hours later, the hospital called and informed us that the patient tested positive for malaria.

Simultaneously, I took a call about a sick traveler from Saudi Arabia. There wasn't Ebola in Saudi Arabia, but there was Middle Eastern Respiratory Syndrome (MERS), the second highly fatal coronavirus that had emerged in 2012. It was to be the third MERS call in recent days and our role was to offer guidance on infection control and arrange testing if indicated. The real work would begin if a patient tested positive, which fortunately had yet to occur. All three patients had other explanations for their symptoms and didn't require testing.

Meanwhile, thirteen campers fell ill with nausea, and several had vomited while waiting on a subway platform after a trip to a community pool. All were transported to a local hospital for evaluation. Group vomiting, especially in kids within a closed space, such as a subway platform, can be psychogenic. One child overdoes it with food, heat, or exertion, and vomits, which triggers others to also lose their lunches. We investigated but could find no other plausible explanation and all the children quickly recovered.

Next came a call from the NYPD's chief surgeon who anxiously reported that two recruits had visited emergency departments for symptoms attributed to viral pericarditis. He wanted to know if there was an outbreak and if we had any intel to share. We did not. While I had him on the phone, I shared that we were once again investigating a report of illegal medical practice. This one involved a person with no medical license or training who was allegedly administering Botox injections. He directed me to call the local precinct.

The week also featured calls about Q fever, a rare disease that is on the list of potential bioterrorism agents; a consult request from Canada on *Mycobacterium marinum* associated with shrimp (we had a *M. marinum* outbreak associated with fish); another consult request from Chicago's health department on meningococcal disease, a child with hand, foot, and mouth disease who lived in a shelter; a complaint about the risk of leptospirosis (more in Chapter 13) from a neighborhood park dog run; and a laboratory call to rule out *Bacillus anthracis* in a patient's blood culture. My desk phone was warm to the touch.

It was a typical week; however, it piled onto an already busy July. Earlier in the month we got a call from colleagues in Pennsylvania who were investigating a report of tetrodotoxin fish poisoning and tracked the possible source back to NYC. Tetrodotoxin is a powerful neurotoxin found in certain fish and can be inadvertently consumed if the fish are incorrectly prepared. The toxin can cause tingling and mouth numbness which may progress to muscle weakness and paralysis. A Pittsburgh area family reportedly purchased puffer fish from a Chinatown fish monger. The father got seriously ill and was placed on a ventilator, the mother was also hospitalized, and the kids had mild symptoms. All recovered and no other illness was uncovered. The foodborne disease unit had tried to locate the fish seller but was also investigating how three nursing home residents had contracted salmonella. This required a joint investigation with our food safety colleagues and the NYS Department of Health, who regulate nursing homes. Oh, and the PHNs were assisting another nursing home with an outbreak of scabies.

Aside from the acute issues, we were in the midst of discussions with the CDC to conduct a study of meningococcal carriage among MSM presenting for sexual health care at a city clinic. It was a follow-up to the 2011–13 outbreak (see Chapter 8). On the non-communicable disease side, the synthetic marijuana compound known as K2 was wreaking havoc again in several neighborhoods by flooding emergency departments with delirious patients. We used our emergency department syndromic surveillance system to monitor this for our colleagues in the Bureau of Alcohol and Drug Use Prevention. Additionally, the syndromic surveillance unit was preparing an annual report of firecracker injuries for the health commissioner. In my spare time, I was preparing a briefing document on the state of illegal medical practice in NYC (see Chapter 10).

We were a little out of breath when on Friday, July 17, 2015, our homegrown automated reportable disease space-time scanning program detected a geographic cluster of eight Legionnaires' disease (LD) reports from the South Bronx. The statistics suggested that a cluster of this size, in these neighborhoods, was only expected to occur once in 500 days. Put a different way, suppose you took an hour-long walk in NYC. Along the way, you found five pennies. Would that strike you as unusual? Probably not. If you took daily hour-long walks in different parts of the city you might find five pennies once every few days. Now suppose you found five, crisp, one-hundred-dollar bills? That would be unusual. You might call it a once-in-a-million-days stroke of good fortune. Furthermore, if you found them all on the same block, you'd probably suspect their presence was related to a common event. Perhaps they fell out of the pocket of a person rushing from the bank. The space-time scanning program mimics how humans use the past to develop an expectation of what is unusual. The other analysis we had in place for LD was more of an alert system. NYC tags every building in the city with a unique identification number, known as the BIN (building identification number). As part of the processing of a new report, the address is mapped to the BIN and then compared to a list of BINs of nursing homes and other congregate settings. A case in such a setting is of high concern because the residents are at higher risk for complications.

Similarly, epidemiologists use communicable disease surveillance data to know when the occurrence of disease is unusual. The analysis compares the number of cases of a disease in space and time to the past to determine the status quo. Five Benjamins found somewhere in the city over thirty days is unusual. On the same block on the same day, extremely unusual. In our example, if those pennies were all from different years and mints, you'd think it was no big deal. But if they all were minted in 2023 from Denver you might suspect a connection. In addition to space (the where) and time (the when), the characteristics (the who) are important to epidemiologists.

Each LD report is assigned to a PHE in the general surveillance unit (GSU) for investigation. The first task is to confirm the diagnosis. *Legionella pneumophila*, the species of the bacterium responsible for most LD infections, is difficult to culture in the lab. Fortunately, there is a urine test that detects a *Legionella* protein to make the diagnosis. The PHE confirms that both the laboratory result and the chest radiograph meet the case criteria. Not every report turns out to be a true LD case, which is one reason why every cluster isn't an outbreak. Late summer and fall are when many LD cases occur and clusters like this one were common, and often didn't turn out to be outbreaks.

LD is caused by *Legionella* species and most often presents as pneumonia. Patients may not have significant cough or phlegm but typically have a fever and headache. Shortness of breath is a worrisome sign, and radiographs of the chest reveal findings like other causes of pneumonia. Gastrointestinal and neurologic complaints don't typically occur with other types of pneumonia but can suggest LD as well as the time of year. Most causes of pneumonia, such as Pneumococcal, occur in cold weather months and are associated with influenza season. LD is a summer/fall illness, although it can occur year-round. *Legionella* are opportunistic infections and victimize the elderly and infirm. Smokers, diabetics, and those with damaged lungs or immune systems are at greatest risk of disease and death, which occurs in about 10% of those infected. Children, unless immunocompromised, are rarely affected. The good news is that there are effective antibiotics to treat LD, and the disease does not spread person-to-person. Exposure to *Legionella* bacteria occurs from environmental sources, universally, man-made devices. The two most common environmental sources are cooling towers and plumbing systems.

Sporadic cases of LD most often don't get tied to a source. However, since *Legionella* can colonize building plumbing systems whenever two or more cases occur in the same building within one year of each other, testing of the plumbing system occurs. The exact exposure isn't always clear, but inhaling shower mist or aspirating drinking water are suspected. Similarly, there are travel LD cases associated with hotel stays that could be due to either the ventilation (as happened at the Bellevue-Stratford Hotel in 1976) or the plumbing system.

There are two parts to the LD case investigation: (1) a patient or proxy interview (2) and a medical chart review. The patient interview seeks to gather the patient's activities in the days before illness onset to uncover possible exposures. Often the patients are too sick to interview, and family members aren't always able to detail their loved one's whereabouts in the ten days before their illness began. Ten days is the range of time from encountering the *Legionella* source to developing symptoms. By retracing a person's steps in that time period, we can get clues as to the location of the source. Typically, it takes the intersection of the paths from multiple people with LD to pinpoint sources, and if multiple LD patients report a common exposure, we call that an outbreak. The second component of LD case investigations involves medical chart reviews which had to be done at the hospital, but now can be done remotely. These are extremely time-consuming, even for staff with expertise. We collect this data to help us understand who is getting ill, to inform prevention messages, and to gain further understanding of disease processes.

In the 1660s, Antoni Van Leeuwenhoek perfected the microscope by improving the invention's ability to magnify small objects 200 times. But it took 200 years before bacteria were fully described and even longer for germ theory to be universally accepted. The genus *Legionella* is a recently discovered scourge, though it likely has been causing disease since the Industrial Revolution expanded urban dwelling. LD was recognized when an outbreak of pneumonia occurred in persons attending the American Legion convention at the Bellevue-Stratford Hotel in Philadelphia in 1976. Large buildings often have central cooling systems that rely on water evaporation to remove heat. Cooling systems play a prominent role in *Legionella* transmission and what sickened 182 and killed 29 people in Philadelphia that bicentennial summer was cross-contamination between the cooling and ventilation systems at the seventy-two-year-old hotel.

Much has been learned since the recognition of *Legionella*. Past outbreaks attributed to the bacterium, discovered retrospectively, date back to 1957 and sources as varied as decorative water fountains to shower heads have been implicated.[98] *Legionella* are found in water, both natural bodies, such as ponds, and human-constructed systems such as building plumbing systems and whirlpools. *Legionella* thrive in warm water and are resistant to levels of chlorine normally used to treat municipal water systems. Humans become exposed to *Legionella* via contaminated aerosols.

Lucretia Jones was the supervisor of the GSU and lived in the Bronx less than a mile from where the *Legionella* cluster was located. Her scared neighbors came to her for information. She was scared too. Lucretia prioritized LD reports, and her staff worked overtime, often heading directly to Bronx hospitals from their homes to review records and speak with patients and their families. The optimal staffing of the GSU was three teams of four PHEs each. At the time we had eight total, but one was still in training, and another was on vacation. One team received twenty-four case assignments the previous week while a member of another team had twenty-three LD cases. They needed help. We reassigned staff from other units to ease the burden and reached out to our sister Bureaus of Tuberculosis and HIV for additional help.

Robert Fitzhenry was the director of the LD unit, which consisted of himself and one other person, and had the task of reviewing the completed investigations to identify commonalities in person, place, or time. It was a tedious process as the chart abstraction and interview forms were extensive. On July 23, Robert wrote and distributed an Epi1 report, a brief situation summary to department leadership and New York State colleagues, on the evolving situation. By Monday, July 27, the LD case count had reached thirty-one in an area of the South Bronx where in the same period in 2013 and 2014 combined there had been five cases.

I scheduled a meeting for the next day to coordinate a department-wide response and to decide whether the Incident Command System (ICS) should be activated. The best way to describe ICS is with a child toy analogy. During regular operations, the health department operates like a car. The different parts have specific functions but with one overall goal: to prevent disease and promote health. Under ICS, the car, like the Transformer toy, reconfigures to become a giant robot, diverting non-essential resources to respond to the emergency. Staff doing similar tasks in different bureaus combine into emergency response groups (ERGs) for efficiency and to maintain continuous operations. The ICS was adapted from the forest fire response model. BCD, along with PHL, Bureau of Public Health Engineering, and the

Communications Office were to take the lead in responding to the LD outbreak with support from the entire agency.

On Tuesday morning, July 28, as I was preparing the agenda for our 1:00 p.m. pre-ICS meeting and noticed among the fifty-plus unopened emails in my inbox one from Alex Gutkovich, a colleague in the NYC Department of Homeless Services. The medical director of a community service organization had notified him of a cluster of pneumonia-like illnesses at a supportive housing facility where they provided medical and social services. Brook House was a six-story building in the Bronx with 190 units, of which 120 housed formerly homeless persons and those living with HIV or AIDS. The email reported that seven residents were ill with suspected pneumonia. I quickly finished the meeting agenda and called the medical director to obtain the patients' names. Two had already been diagnosed with LD and had been detected by the BIN analysis earlier that morning. The others were assigned to staff for follow-up. I made a mental note of the address of Brook House, 455 E. 148th Street.

We felt the urgency to find and decontaminate the source. The NY Wadsworth Center Laboratory, located in Albany, is one of the best public health labs in the country, and the chief of bacterial diseases at the time, Kimberlee Musser, was an ally we could rely on. In 2014, the Wadsworth Center deployed a new technology during an LD outbreak in a different part of the Bronx. Co-op City is a thirty-five-building high-rise development that was built in the 1960s and 1970s in the northeast Bronx adjacent to the Hutchinson River. Eight cases of LD occurred in Co-op City residents in November and December 2014. With the assistance of the Wadsworth Center's in-house developed PCR test for *Legionella* DNA, the source was traced to the power plant cooling tower. The PCR test could be used on environmental water and swab samples and was a tremendous advancement that allowed public health investigators to rapidly evaluate sources. The Wadsworth PCR test could distinguish three levels of specificity: *Legionella, Legionella pneumophila* (Lp), and *Legionella pneumophila* type 1 (Lp1). Lp1 is the most common strain that causes outbreaks.

During the pre-ICS meeting, we established boundaries for the outbreak zone using the zip codes of the cases to focus environmental sampling. The geography of cases made a single plumbing system impossible and multiple simultaneous plumbing systems causing LD had never happened. It had to be a cooling tower, but where were the cooling towers? In 2015 there was no system in NYC to keep track of cooling towers. Our environmental counterparts from Public Health Engineering (PHEng) shared that there were two incomplete sources. The NYC Department of Environmental Protection knew of businesses that had applied for sewer credits since the cooling tower water was recycled and not discharged into the sewer system. The NYC Department of Buildings (DOB) also had a list of new construction permits that included the installation of a cooling tower. PHEng staff also searched for cooling towers on foot and with satellite imagery. Rodolfo Perez from PHEng was tasked with merging the two partial lists to create a map of the cooling towers. For testing, it was decided for the greatest efficiency that samples would be split. Wadsworth would do the rapid PCR and our PHL would follow up and culture those that were positive by PCR for *Legionella pneumophila*, including Lp1. The department's Health Police offered to drive the samples to Albany. At the time it seemed like a reasonable plan and use of resources. Sampling would begin that evening.

After the meeting, I returned to my desk and studied the

map of case locations. They were spread among seven South Bronx zip codes in the neighborhoods of High Bridge, Hunts Point, Morrisania, and Mott Haven. East 149th Street is the main east–west thoroughfare in the South Bronx. On the west end is Lincoln Hospital and on the east end is St. Mary's Park. The cases' residences were mostly distributed on either side of E. 149th Street beginning at the hospital and stretching past the park as if sprayed from a fire hose. The greatest concentration of cases was south of 149th Street and just west of St. Mary's Park.

Robert had shown me what a cooling tower looked like from satellite imagery; essentially the cylindrical blades of a fan in a rectangular structure that was larger than an exhaust fan. I brought up the satellite image of E. 149th Street in the South Bronx and began scanning slowly at the highest magnification. I reasoned that since the prevailing winds blew west to east, I should start at St. Ann's Street, just west of the park, and track west. I inched along, scanning a block north and south of E. 149th Street as if zigzagging through squares on a chess board. I saw small fan blades, often in pairs or quads, but nothing large enough to suspect a cooling tower. I crossed Brook Avenue. Then, at 436-440 E 149th Street I spied a single, four-blade fan in a metallic-looking rectangular enclosure that was five times larger than all the others I had seen. It was located at the rear of the roof. I pulled Robert away from his case reviews and he confirmed my suspicion. The cooling tower was located at the address of a hotel and gym.

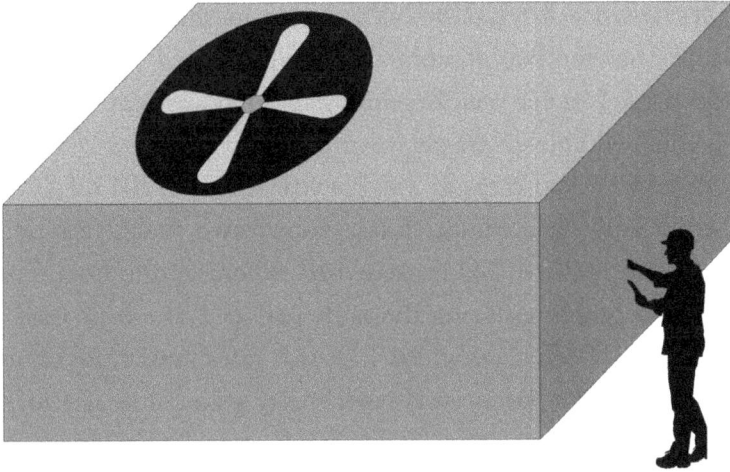

Representation of the four-blade fan device seen on roof at 436 East 149th Street, Bronx, NY on July 28, 2015

Rodolfo shared the map of the cooling towers in the South Bronx culled from city records. Sixteen red dots represented the cooling towers and stretched the width of the Bronx from E. 138th Street north to Yankee Stadium. I placed Rodolfo's map next to the case map on my dual video display screens. Only four cooling towers on Rodolfo's map were proximate to the cluster of cases to be the potential source. The multiple cooling towers on top of Lincoln Hospital were worrisome suspects as was a Verizon facility a block or two further east on 150th Street. The cooling tower I had found was not present on Rodolfo's map. Inspectors with sampling kits had already been dispatched to six sites with single or multiple cooling towers. The city lab was told to expect samples after 10 p.m. Wadsworth would receive their samples well after midnight. I called Chris Boyd, the director of PHEng who was overseeing the environmental sampling operation. I asked about the cooling tower at 436-440 E. 149th Street, but it was too late to add it to the day's sampling. It would have to wait another day.

Surveillance for LD in NYC began in the 1980s. For two decades the number of annual cases fluctuated but remained between 10–100 per year. Beginning in 2006, case counts topped and remained above 100 per year. By the end of the 2010s, the LD case count had crept to 200 per year. Then, in 2013, LD took off, increasing by a hundred cases every two years, reaching a peak of 656 in 2018. LD increased elsewhere on the East Coast, more than doubling during the same period. Europe also saw an increase. In NYC, the highest LD case rates are in the poorest communities. The Bronx was particularly vulnerable, not just in terms of poverty, but because of its high rates of chronic diseases including asthma, diabetes, and HIV.

We'd been chasing community outbreaks of LD since the early 2000s. In 2006, former DOD and LD epidemiologist Dan Cimini became concerned about cases in the Northeast Bronx. Twenty-nine LD cases had occurred in and around the Parkchester housing complex over a five-month period. Dan directed the GSU to ask patients about their work, commuting, and where they shopped and recreated. No common links stood out. He walked the neighborhood, practicing shoe-leather epidemiology, looking for rooftop cooling towers and other aerosol water sources. Grocery store misters were considered. A decorative fountain in the apartment complex became a suspect. Since no cultures were obtained from any patient there was nothing to compare to environmental cultures, so no samples were collected, and the outbreak went unsolved. Six years later, two more LD cases occurred in the same apartment complex. PHE Renee Pouchet learned that the two men had spent time near the fountain. This time, the fountain was sampled but no *Legionella* was recovered. No additional LD cases were found at the apartment complex, and we moved on to other outbreaks.

Central air conditioning systems employ chiller systems employing water to cool air. The temperature of municipal tap water in NYC averages 54°F. As the water passes through pipes in the chiller system, heat is exchanged—the warmer air (75°F) is cooled by passing over an array of pipes carrying the cold water. The water warms and cooling towers are employed to exchange the heat picked up by the water into the atmosphere. While the water in the chiller system is in a closed loop, the water used in cooling towers is separate and in an open-air device. Water is then sprayed down a column of coiled pipes to cool the chiller system's water. The sprayed water is subsequently collected in a pan at the bottom of the tower and pumped back up to the spray devices at the top. Fans are employed to draw air upward, and in this process, water evaporates, then releasing heat, which cools the water in the pipes (see diagram).

It is not a perfect system and vapor escapes from the top. If not treated sufficiently with disinfectants, *Legionella* can grow in the water in the collecting pan at the base of the cooling tower and be expelled out the top of the tower. Biocides, chemicals used to kill bacteria and other organisms, are added to the water. Too little is ineffective and too much corrodes the pan and pipes. Automatic systems have been designed to add biocide at regular intervals. Alarms notify when biocide supply levels are low, but despite safeguards, cooling tower maintenance is anything but routine. Evaporative cooling towers are typically placed on the roofs of buildings and should not be confused with water towers, the barrel-shaped tanks often seen on NYC rooftops from street level.

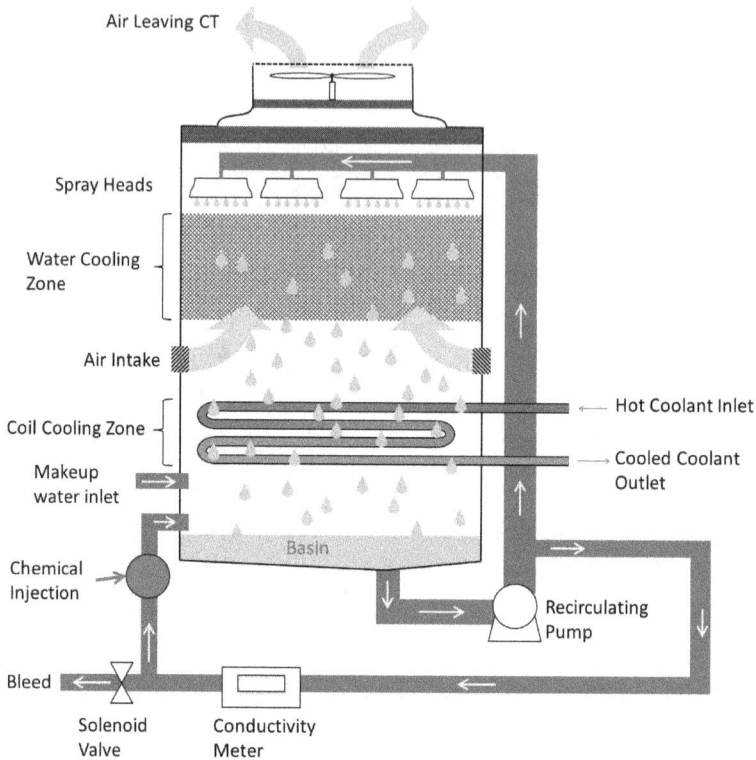

Diagram of a Cooling Tower, courtesy of Rodolfo Perez, PhD

What has caused the increase in LD is largely unknown. Some of the rise may be due to greater awareness and testing, and some might be due to the increased use of cooling towers, but there's little data on how this industry has expanded in the past several decades. Fortune Business Insights, a financial consulting firm, estimates that the global cooling tower market will grow from $3.82 billion to $5.29 billion by the end of the decade.[99] There are an estimated 2 million cooling towers in the United States in 2024,[100] but how many were there in 2015? Registration of cooling towers in NYC began at the end of 2015. By November

2016 there were 4,806 systems registered. In 2024, the latest data published, the number reached 6,008.[101] Part of the increase could be delayed registration, but there are fines for failing to register so this 25% increase over eight years seems real. I recall looking out the window of our Long Island City office and spotting cooling towers on the top of new buildings. There was even a trailer parked on Twenty-Eighth Street in Long Island City with a brand-new cooling tower waiting to be hoisted to the roof of the building under construction across the street from our offices.

By the end of the twenty-first century, cooling towers were proven to be a major source of aerosolized *Legionella*. In the town of Murcia, Spain, over 400 LD cases were attributed to a hospital cooling tower.[102] The position of the tower allowed transmission of LD up to three-quarters of a mile away. Melbourne, Australia experienced an outbreak in 2000 in visitors to the aquarium. The newly installed cooling tower exhaust was forty-six feet above ground level and was responsible for 125 cases.[103] In the town of Barrow-in-Furness, England, the town's arts center sickened 494, with 180 laboratory-confirmed LD infections.[104] Only one of the two cooling towers was operational and was located on the third level of the car park. Among several errors, the biocide container, responsible for disinfecting the cooling tower water, was empty. You get the idea. Outbreaks, especially large ones, are associated with inadequately operated or maintained cooling towers. The closer to the ground the cooling tower is, the greater the risk for LD.

It was the November 2014 outbreak that occurred in Portugal that grabbed the attention of Dr. Sharon Balter, who was the supervisor of the foodborne and waterborne units. A cooling tower from a factory spread *Legionella* throughout the suburbs of Lisbon infecting 377 people and killing fourteen.[105] An exceptionally warm fall and a thermal inversion were cited as contributory factors. Sharon became concerned about what this meant for NYC and sought to put in place building regulations, but her efforts met resistance and stalled.

Underlying the concern over cooling towers, which serve as both a reservoir and amplification vehicle for *Legionella*, is global warming. *Legionella* thrive in warm, wet climates. Global warming has created the ideal climate for *Legionella* growth by elevating temperatures and redistributing water. Here in the States, particularly East Coast cities, with their concentration of concrete and steel, have gotten warmer necessitating greater need and use of air conditioning systems. The increase in LD cases over the past twenty years parallels the warming of our planet.

I was born in the Bronx, as were my parents. But I didn't live in the Bronx until many years later during my pediatric residency. My family lived across the East River in the northern Manhattan neighborhood called Inwood. I recall trips to visit my cousins in Long Island and how we would pass through the Bronx on the South Bronx Expressway. I'd look out the window at the rows of vacant shells of burned-out tenement buildings and wonder what had happened to them. In the 1950s, public housing was built in the South Bronx while more luxury high-rise apartments were built farther north in Riverdale. Urban renewal forced many low-income Manhattan residents to move north to the Bronx where they could afford the rents. Rent control squeezed landlords who couldn't afford the upkeep and taxes on their buildings. The fires were quite possibly the result of arson. City policies at the time allowed tenants who experienced a fire to get housing assistance and reimbursement for lost possessions. Could this have been an incentive to burn? In the 1980s and 1990s, new housing was built in the Bronx and businesses returned, perhaps bringing with them cooling towers. Despite having some of the wealthiest communities in the city, the Bronx has been and remains the poorest county in the state of New York, and South Bronx neighborhoods lead NYC in the rates of diabetes and HIV.

It hasn't always been this way. For most of the nineteenth and twentieth centuries, the Bronx was a vibrant and thriving borough, and home to hard-working immigrants. It boasted parks, universities, a zoo, and a botanical garden. In 1904, the first subway connecting the Bronx to Manhattan opened. Perennial World Series champions, the New York Yankees, moved into their new stadium in the Bronx in 1923. New five and six-story apartment buildings rose like mushrooms and unlike most dwellings of prewar NYC, the apartments had private bathrooms and central heating. The Metropolitan Life Insurance Company built Parkchester, a novel housing development on sixty-six acres in the East Bronx, essentially a city within the city. Over 12,000 units were created along with a shopping center, parks, playgrounds, and grocery stores. It had a centralized plant to provide heat and hot water, a trend that would later have implications for LD. When another wave of immigrants seeking opportunity moved to NYC in the 1960s and 70s, and additional housing was needed, the holistic Parkchester model wasn't followed. The housing constructed was dense, soulless, high-rise buildings without the same support systems and community amenities.

My father grew up a few blocks from Yankee Stadium on the Grand Concourse, a magnificent thoroughfare with a park between the north and southbound roadways. A dozen blocks south, E. 149th Street was a bustling economic hub with department stores, restaurants, movie and vaudeville theaters, as well as an opera house. The Bronx Opera House opened in 1913 at 436 E. 149th Street and showcased stars and acts as varied as

Fats Waller, Harry Houdini, Lionel and Ethel Barrymore, and the Marx Brothers. And there were operas too: *Aida, Carmen, Madam Butterfly, and Hansel and Gretel*, all in English, highlighted the 1916 season. Over the ensuing decades, the opera house served as a movie theater and church, eventually reincarnating as the Opera House Hotel which opened in 2013.

The cooling tower I had spied on satellite imagery was on the roof of the Opera House Hotel. I navigated to their website where the landing page had a photo of the hotel taken at night with the facade lit by footlights, like a stage. It didn't look big, maybe four stories high, and offered sixty rooms and conference space occupying less than a city block. The rooms looked fancy in a way that was both modern and a throwback to a bygone era. I mapped 455 E. 148th Street, the Brook House, where there was a cluster of pneumonia cases. The building loomed just behind the Opera House Hotel to the east on an adjacent lot. I would later see a photograph taken from Brook House's third-floor patio that had a direct view of the roof of the Opera House Hotel. The CDC emailed us on Wednesday, July 30, 2015, to share that the North Carolina Health Department had an LD case in one of their residents who had traveled to NYC before the illness onset. The person had stayed at the Opera House Hotel.

Brook House staff went door-to-door to perform wellness checks on their residents. On the third floor, one resident didn't answer. The tenant was sixty-nine years old and kept mostly to himself. Staff knew little of his medical history, his comings and goings, or if he had been ill. The last contact anyone could recall with him had been two weeks earlier. When staff gained access to his room, he was found dead. By this point, we knew of two confirmed LD deaths connected to the South Bronx outbreak. Deaths in LD outbreaks, as with most outbreaks, lag behind case counts. Case reporting occurs electronically by laboratories and is relatively timely. Deaths occur days to weeks after diagnosis and require either an epidemiologist to follow up with hospitals or for the death certificate to be filed with the Office of Vital Statistics (OVS) listing LD as the cause of death. I connected with OVS and had them set up a surveillance system for LD deaths. Next, I reached out to the OCME to enlist their help in examining and diagnosing Bronx deaths suspicious of LD. The first referral to the OCME was from Brook House. Kim at the Wadsworth Center agreed to test postmortem samples.

We also had our PHEs call all the hospitals in the Bronx and Northern Manhattan to ask them to assist in the investigation by instructing their staff to suspect LD, submit any existing patient cultures to the PHL as well as obtain culture specimens on new patients, notify us if a patient died, and facilitate our efforts to conduct chart reviews. The information was also shared in a health alert to inform the medical community. Patient culture specimens are a critical component in connecting LD outbreaks to environmental sources. This is where DNA and molecular epidemiology shine. Like matching a crime suspect's DNA to the victim and crime scene, we match DNA from patients to the suspected source—in this case, one or more cooling towers.

On July 30, while we awaited the first cooling tower results, Robert accompanied the environmental team to the Opera House Hotel. He emailed back confirming that what we saw on the satellite image was indeed a cooling tower. It looked new and well maintained, but that was not a reliable predictor of *Legionella* results, and samples were obtained. Sampling included water chemistries including residual chlorine, a measure of available disinfectant. There was no measurable residual chlorine in the cooling tower water sample from the Opera House Hotel.

I next plotted the location of the Opera House Hotel on the LD case map. Cases clustered around it, especially to the east and south. Other sites sampled on day two of the environmental investigation included two additional cooling towers at Lincoln Hospital, the Verizon facility, and two buildings near Yankee Stadium and the Grand Concourse. The LD case count was now sixty-seven. The first set of cooling tower *Legionella* results came back just after 4 p.m. on July 29. Four locations had been accessed and sampled. Two locations were positive for Lp1—a building on 161st Street near the courthouse and a Lincoln Hospital cooling tower—though the PCR signal from the latter was weak. It would take days to a week to grow *Legionella* in the lab, the next step toward linking the source to patients. However, the Commissioner's orders didn't need to wait for these results and were immediately issued to building owners to disinfect the cooling tower.

If you've ever read a contemporary, true or fictional, crime story, you know about DNA. To implicate a person in a crime, the police need a DNA sample from the crime scene and one from the suspect. The two samples are sequenced, and analogous sections (alleles) are compared. The more alleles used in the comparison the greater confidence the police have that a match is real and not a coincidence. Without DNA samples from both the crime scene and the suspect, the technique can't be used. Analogously, for molecular epidemiology to implicate an environmental source in a patient infection we need a *Legionella* culture from both. The crime and disease techniques aren't exactly the same. For one, bacteria have far smaller genomes than humans so instead of looking at a dozen or so alleles it is possible to examine the entire genome. And while human genomes differ, except for identical siblings, those of bacteria can be conserved.

Bacteria multiply by cell division creating two identical daughter cells. Some bacteria mutate quickly, such that those daughter cells if exposed to different environments diverge genetically and are no longer identical. While others mutate more slowly and remain indistinguishable genetically for some time. So, the collection time matters. However, the most difficult obstacle to overcome in using molecular epidemiology to identify sources of LD outbreaks is due to the nature of *Legionella*. Human specimen collection is difficult because patients often don't have productive coughs. Furthermore, the bacterium is hard to grow in the laboratory and requires special nutrients. Finally, medical providers treat pneumonia empirically, meaning they decide on treatment without obtaining a culture test.

Molecular epidemiology techniques were evolving at the time of the outbreak, and three methods were employed. In order of their discriminatory power were: PFGE, sequence-based typing (SBT), and WGS. Two *Legionella* isolates could have the same PFGE and SBT patterns but still have different WGS sequences. While all the results were of interest academically, only WGS was relied upon to pinpoint the source.

We worked long hours during outbreaks, especially in the initial days, often losing track of time and skipping meals. I sent an email just after 7 p.m. on July 29 to my boss, Assistant Commissioner Dr. Marci Layton, and her boss, Deputy Commissioner and ICS Incident Commander Dr. Jay Varma, and Deputy Commissioner for Environmental Health Dan Kass, laying out the evidence that led me to believe that the Opera House Hotel cooling tower was responsible and that we needed to shut it down since it could not yet be ordered to disinfect. The PCR result wouldn't be back for another twenty-four hours or so, and while we had a positive result from Lincoln Hospital, the clustering of cases, the proximity of the cooling tower to street level, cases at Brook House, and the case in a guest of the hotel without another cooling tower in the immediate vicinity, convinced me we had found the source. Because nighttime temperatures had been in the high 70s, shutting off the hotel cooling tower would mean shutting off the air conditioning and relocating all the guests. My arguments were persuasive, but we lacked the proof needed to issue such an order. For all we knew there could still be unknown cooling towers in the neighborhood, or it could still be the hospital cooling tower.

That summer marked my fifteenth year with the department, and I had already been through dozens of outbreaks, big and small, and had worked under four health commissioners and three mayors. There had been numerous emotionally and politically charged outbreaks. The anthrax letters, SARS, meningococcal outbreaks in substance users and gay men, the emergence of novel H1N1 influenza, and a case of imported Ebola virus all raised the level of anxiety in NYC to unprecedented heights, but we at the health department had always been viewed and treated as professionals, first responders, and allies in the fight. We were the experts, having earned our D❂D moniker. *Legionella* changed all that.

I don't recall exactly when it started, but Governor Andrew Cuomo and Mayor Bill de Blasio engaged in a wrestling match to rival the theatrics of WWE. They fought to be the first to announce new cases and deaths. Cuomo sent teams to the Bronx to search door-to-door for cooling towers. De Blasio responded by demanding that 500 staff be reassigned and trained to be inspectors. If de Blasio held press conferences at 1:00 p.m., Cuomo moved his to 11:00 a.m. Public health practitioners on each side were caught in the middle. We had always worked together, but we now were instructed to not share information. Since the Wadsworth Center was doing the PCR tests on cooling towers,

Cuomo had an advantage. Is this what set de Blasio against his own health department? Or was it that we made decisions based on data and not optics?

Mayor Bloomberg tabbed Tom Frieden to be health commissioner in 2003 and then moved on to economic issues that were his priority. He enabled the agency leaders he had selected to perform their jobs. Frieden was confident, assertive, and vocal. Under his leadership, the department became ever more autonomous, and data driven. We had accumulated a cadre of experienced public health practitioners who had expertise and had earned international and national recognition. Frieden did his job and Bloomberg respected us enough to leave us alone. During the seven years Frieden was health commissioner (2002–2009), we had a few large communicable disease events. The original SARS virus burst on the scene in the winter of 2002, and although there were no cases in NYC, we were consumed with preparation and surveillance for most of 2003. A single case of inhalation anthrax was traced to imported animal hides used to make drums in early 2006 and was followed soon after by a meningococcal outbreak (detailed in Chapter 8). In 2009, a novel influenza strain emerged and circled the globe raising the specter of the 1918 pandemic, causing school closures and public anxiety. The approach to these public health threats was methodical, science-based, and led by the health department. Tom Frieden left the department in 2009 to become CDC director, and Mayor Bloomberg chose Mary Bassett as his successor. Bassett was less visible than Frieden, yet as competent and thrived seamlessly under the Bloomberg system.

Bill de Blasio started his tenure as mayor in 2014 and immediately sought to distinguish himself from his predecessor. De Blasio, who had been the public advocate, fashioned himself as a man of the people who didn't hesitate to criticize the government, specifically his own agencies. The wheels of government would move quicker under his watch and bureaucracy was a target. We all want less red tape. De Blasio reminded administrators that he had been elected by the people, and therefore owned the responsibility of all aspects of government. Department leadership, accustomed to having their expertise and decision-making authority respected, soon came into conflict with the mayor. The first clash came at a meeting before a press conference announcing the results of *Legionella* testing at Lincoln Hospital attended by various commissioners and deputies of city agencies, including the health department.

De Blasio didn't appear to absorb or accept information from the health department well. When he was told that there was no registry of cooling towers, he was incredulous and lashed out at the department with a barrage of curses and name-calling as was relayed to me by a high-ranking health department official in the meeting. It didn't matter that such a registry didn't exist anywhere in the United States. When the nature and course of LD were explained to him, he responded by pointing a finger and chastising that our problem was that we knew too much. I was told that de Blasio said we should stick to the science and leave the communication to him because he was the expert. The implication, to myself and departmental colleagues, was that our knowledge was worthless in the face of a crisis. Because of LD's incubation period—the time from exposure to the source until the beginning of symptoms—that could be as long as ten to fourteen days, we could expect that even after we identified and disinfected the source or sources, there would continue to be new cases. This news, despite supportive evidence provided by others including the CDC, was not acceptable to Mayor de Blasio. When presented with a plan to prioritize cooling towers in the South Bronx he ordered us to do the entire city. When Willie Sutton, the noted gangster, was asked why he robbed banks he responded, "That's where the money is." The health department's plan was to use data to narrow the search to find the offending cooling tower quickly. Instead, we were told to spread resources thinly over the entire city. It made little sense during an acute outbreak and appeared optics driven.

To borrow a phrase from autocrats and gamblers, the mayor doubled down. When he was presented with an estimate of the resources and time it would take to accomplish a citywide search, inspection, and remediation of all cooling towers, de Blasio proceeded to order the use of all the city's resources and demanded the work be completed in two weeks. He also made a point of reminding department leadership that this wasn't the Bloomberg administration. This marked the beginning of a contentious relationship that would last his entire administration.

Deputy Commissioner for Environmental Health Dan Kass, who was in the room for this initial meeting, described it as panic, and what ensued as chaos. The governor made things worse when he clashed with the mayor claiming City agencies couldn't handle the crisis. State agencies in turn sent their own team into NYC to find cooling towers. Both Cuomo and de Blasio publicly appeared to be cooperating, but behind the media lights they instructed state and city workers from collaborating, but we did anyway, just out of their view. It was the only tactical way to approach the problem.

De Blasio believed, not unreasonably, that bureaucracy can impede getting things done. I doubt anyone would argue with that, but his style of distrusting and berating staff was not productive. If you keep beating your pack horse, you will soon be traveling alone. It made the stress of the situation imminently worse. Identifying and inspecting every cooling tower in the city required massive resources, beyond the health and buildings departments, but also the police and fire departments. De Blasio also accepted no excuse not to gain access to a building. Dan had conversations with the health department's general counsel who clearly advised that the department did not have the legal authority to enter a building without permission. Furthermore, cooling towers weren't toys—if not approached with care by knowledgeable staff—injuries could result. Especially after dark.

At another meeting, this one at City Hall, the mayor was over ninety minutes late. An unfortunate official mistimed his trip to the restroom and returned to the conference room after de Blasio had made his appearance. He promptly was reamed out for being late. No one came to his defense, they just looked across the table at each other with knowing eyes. The task of identifying every cooling tower was not completed, and the mayor ordered staff to work around the clock. The mayor then called on each agency, one by one, and each administrator fearing admonishment replied, no problem. Until he got to the health department. Dan attempted to explain that we couldn't legally enter without the owner's permission and that examining a cooling tower at night without a person who knew how it operated was dangerous to staff. The situation wasn't equivalent to a fire or a known criminal harbored inside. There simply wasn't the risk to justify. As you might expect, that didn't go over well. The city would do this with or without the health department.

The understanding of risk, as esoteric as it sounds, was a critical issue. In public health, risk is on a continuum. Your risk of getting lung cancer rises with the number of packs of cigarettes and years you smoke. Data drives the mitigation of risk to yield the greatest benefit. As a result, hard choices are common. Harm reduction using needle exchange is an example. Intravenous drug use has many risks, but by itself, as a public health issue, it cannot be simply mitigated. But, by removing contaminated needles from being shared we can reduce the risk of several serious infectious diseases. The mayor appeared to view risk as dichotomous, it was either present or it wasn't. If risk was present, the solution was to throw every resource at it to mitigate the hell out of it. That might be fine if you have only one risk to deal with or have unlimited, renewable resources, or if the risk is to your very existence—think of the war in Ukraine.

Late one night, early in the response, a team of health inspectors, firefighters, and police officers knocked on the door of a building. There was no answer. The firefighters took an axe and broke down the door. The inspectors were ordered to the roof. The inspectors refused and called back to their supervisors who confirmed with Dan and the health commissioner that they should not enter. This quickly got back to the Mayor's Office and Dan soon was called by a city official who screamed and ordered him to send his staff into the building. Dan calmly tried to present the legal reasons why he couldn't, but the official would have none of it. Likely, Dan had been yelled at by someone, who themselves had been yelled at by a staffer in the mayor's chain of abuse. Dan was again ordered to send the inspectors to the roof. Dan politely refused. Not only was it illegal, but it also wasn't safe. Several months later, after the LD outbreak had ended, the health commissioner was allegedly told to fire Dan. She politely refused.

While de Blasio praised the D❂Ds in public, snapping photos with them at press events, out of the view of cameras and microphones, my experience was that he and his staff were bullies. He blamed us, the messengers, for the outbreak and questioned the speed of our response. Poverty and poor health in the Bronx were problems that multiple administrations had failed to remedy. Was he angered that early in the outbreak epidemiologists used zip code boundaries to define the outbreak area, while the environmental group used a slightly different impact boundary for deciding where to test? Perhaps his ire was triggered because case numbers reported by the State didn't always agree with our numbers, generating media questions. A representative of the Mayor's Office demanded that we round up all the data technicians who touch the data and get them all in a room with data on the screen and await further instructions. A request that, to me, rang of fascism. The meeting never happened, but the Mayor's Office sent a twenty-something aide, who demonstrated miniscule understanding of statistics or epidemiology, to stand menacingly behind staff while they updated the case maps. He periodically called back to his bosses and instructed us on the exact shade of green preferred. Two days later he was gone.

The sample from the Opera House Hotel was strongly positive for Lp1. I'm not sure if Dan Kass knew this when he was called to City Hall, but we were confident early on that we had found the source. The hotel was ordered to disinfect which was completed by their contractor on August 1. The cooling tower was operational six months of the year, from May until October. Examination of the cooling tower and maintenance records revealed the use of an automatic system to inject the biocide. The injection was to occur once a day but was contingent upon the pump being on to circulate the water. This was a precaution to prevent corrosion. The pump was in turn controlled by a thermoregulator that turned on when the entering coolant temperature was 87°F or higher. The biocide reservoir holds ten gallons and was set to inject once daily; therefore, biocide consumption was approximately one gallon per month. Records show that the tank was filled on May 4, 2014.

Three months later, two more gallons were added. Biocide wasn't added again until July 21, 2015, when two gallons were added. A few weeks later in August, the tank needed nine gallons. Five more gallons were added a week later. The tanks were not opaque, so the level could not be easily assessed. The low chlorine residual and growth of *Legionella* detected on July 30, 2015, strongly suggested that the automatically added biocide was insufficient. In ensuing weeks, the biocide frequency was increased to twice daily and the chlorine residual remained low resulting in a third daily biocide injection. We could not ascertain if the biocide injections failed to occur because the water circulation pump wasn't triggered, but this would explain why only two gallons were needed between May 2014 and July 2015.

Aside from Brook House there were a few other locations where LD cases occurred that had us worried. Several cases occurred at a nursing home 1.3 miles north of the main cluster of cases. Residents were said to be fond of sitting outdoors and this could've increased their exposure to contaminated mist. But was the mist from the Opera House Hotel cooling tower or another source? Cases were also found closer to the epicenter in the Melrose Houses, nine public housing buildings operated by the NYC Housing Authority.

Two or more cases in the same building triggers an evaluation of the potable water system. *Legionella* can survive in plumbing systems, preferring the hot water side and dead legs. Plumbing dead legs are pipes that receive little or intermittent water flow. Biofilms can grow and support *Legionella* colonization. Bacteria can then dislodge, enter apartments, and expose residents through faucets and shower heads. You might think that with the preponderance of evidence suggesting that community, and not building transmission was occurring, testing would be deemed unnecessary.

Not so. Politics being what they are, this was not acceptable. And while it was highly unlikely for there to have been overlapping community and building sources in the same community, testing proceeded of the Melrose plumbing system out of an abundance of caution. Nothing was found but, pardon the pun, it drained additional departmental resources.

The search for cooling towers continued. While we wished to focus on the South Bronx, political pressure forced us to expand to other boroughs. This placed enormous stress on the laboratories and environmental staff and created delays. To make matters worse, the inspectors reassigned were neglecting their other duties, such as restaurant and building inspections.

Nonetheless, proving the LD outbreak source proceeded in a stepwise fashion that exploited the advances in bacterial genomics. The first level of suspicion came from a positive cooling tower PCR sample for Lp1. Positive samples then were cultured on specialized *Legionella* growth media. After five to seven days, if the culture was positive there would be sufficient growth to move on to the next steps: SBT and PFGE. Both methods use parts of the bacterial genome to characterize and differentiate strains. Like using a witness's description of hair color, eye color, height, and weight to characterize a bank robber, the methods can narrow down the list of suspects, but not perfectly identify the culprit. Simultaneously, samples were prepared for the gold-standard test: WGS. Because samples were collected over several weeks, the laboratory work-up periods for the dozens of cooling towers in the South Bronx overlapped, like the weeks of employees' summer vacations. The answer could only be revealed with certainty once all the testing was completed.

Fifty-five cooling towers were tested in the South Bronx outbreak zone, with twenty-one found to have Lp1 by PCR. Fourteen were able to be cultured and both PFGE and SBT agreed that two cooling tower *Legionella* isolates matched patient isolates. We could have gotten lucky and had only one match. Conversely, six could've matched. We needed to await WGS for our answer. It was midway through August when all the testing was complete.

The unit of comparison in WGS is called a single nucleotide polymorphism (SNP). DNA is made up of four distinct nucleotides: adenine (A), cytosine (C), guanine (G), and thymine (T). The nucleotides are attached in a chain; the exact order uniquely characterizes the sample. Often a DNA gene is represented like this: CTG ACT GTG GAG AAG TCT. This sequence is part of the gene for hemoglobin S, the mutant form that causes sickle cell anemia. The analogous sequence for the normal version, hemoglobin A, is: CTG ACT GAG GAG AAG TCT. Notice the difference? Three sequential nucleotides are called a codon and the third codon in the sickle cell sequence has been altered by a single nucleotide (A->T). That's a SNP.

The two sites that had matching patterns on PFGE and SBT were the Opera House Hotel and Pyramid Safe House, a shelter. The Pyramid Safe House was farther north in the Bronx and was not supported as the source by the epidemiology. There were no cases in either the shelter residents or staff. Cases didn't cluster around the building or report exposure to the shelter. The isolate from the shelter differed by a single nucleotide from the Opera House Hotel. Twenty-six patient isolates had the same WGS sequence and matched to only one cooling tower, the Opera House Hotel.

This strain was not new. In the archive were five previous patients dating back to 2010. It took two weeks from collecting samples from the Opera House Hotel to matching the genetic sequence to the twenty-six patients. But it took another week to complete the same analysis on all the other Lp1 positive cooling towers to establish that the hotel, and only the hotel, was responsible for the outbreak. On August 20, the City declared the outbreak over and the mystery solved. The last patient became ill on August 3. All in all, 138 people had become ill and sixteen died, five of whom were found dead at home. The actual number of cases was likely higher, as LD is often missed, especially in persons who have a milder illness.

Upon our return visit to the Opera House Hotel's cooling tower, the chlorine residual was again zero and the water was positive for Lp1, so further remediation was instructed. At the conclusion of our investigation, the evidence implicating the Opera House Hotel cooling tower as the source of the outbreak included two guests contracting LD after their stay, three LD cases in neighboring Brook House residents, the clustering around the hotel was statistically significant, the cooling tower was repeatedly found to be positive for Lp1, and the most damning of all—twenty-six patients' cultures matched by WGS to the isolate from the hotel.

But there was still a loose end to tie. One of the patients whose isolate matched the Opera House Hotel strain lived five miles away in the North Bronx. He reported working in Manhattan and had told the initial interviewer that he spent no time in the exposure zone. I reinterviewed him and asked him how he got to work every day. He didn't own a car so took two buses. He waited for the bus transfer on E. 149th Street, one block from the Opera House Hotel.

The Bronx has repeatedly been the site of LD cases and outbreaks. While data on chronic health conditions support the assertion that Bronx residents are likely more susceptible, there's more to the story. An analysis found that the median height of cooling towers in the Bronx was four stories while in Manhattan it is fourteen stories. Proximity to ground level in densely populated areas is a risk. To mitigate future LD disease and prevent outbreaks, several laws were passed. Registration and maintenance of cooling towers became a requirement along with regular inspection and testing for *Legionella*. Reporting of positive results is to be made to the health department, and corrective action of positive results and follow-up are spelled out in the regulations.

We had hardly caught our breath when another *Legionella* cluster surfaced, this time it was three cases in the same Northeast Bronx zip code. Renee Pouchet recognized that a patient's work address and another's home address were on the same block. We were off running again.

CHAPTER 13

Muerto Vivero

T'was days before Christmas, two-thousand sixteen,
The city was humming, the streets were unclean.
Creatures were stirring, scurrying hither and yon,
Where heaps of trash lay waiting, the rats feasted on.

There's a famous meme based on a 2015 video showing a rat dragging an uneaten pizza slice down NYC subway stairs. As any New Yorker will tell you, rats are ubiquitous in the city. Pass a garbage bag on the street and you shouldn't be surprised when it moves. Unlike their urban neighbor, the pigeon, rats prefer to go unnoticed, so it was a bit unusual that Pizza Rat was captured on the several-second video. Rats historically are associated with disease, most notably the Bubonic plague which killed 20 million people in Europe in the 1350s. But the Black Death was a long time ago, and society and urban landscapes have changed. Rats avoid humans, we have better sanitation, so how can they be the source of disease in NYC?

One year to the day that Pizza Rat first appeared on the internet we received a call from a hospital infection control practitioner. Dr. Daniel Eiras, who would later join the health department during COVID-19, reported an unknown illness in a middle-aged man. The man, who I'll call Mr. Santiago, became ill on December 16 with chills and muscle aches in his thighs. He developed a low-grade fever along with diarrhea and generalized weakness. Upon reaching the hospital he was noted to have jaundice, a yellowing of the skin indicative of liver failure. Additionally, both his platelets, a key component of the blood clotting system, and oxygen levels, were low. He rapidly developed kidney failure and respiratory distress and required life support.

Mr. Santiago was in the intensive care unit, sedated, and on a ventilator. His physicians were scrambling to diagnose and treat him. This specific constellation of triple organ damage—liver, kidney, respiratory—brought to their minds leptospirosis. The man resided in Brooklyn, but a key clue was that he worked at a vivero in the Bronx. We were familiar with viveros, live animal markets that allow consumers to select a chicken, rabbit, goat, or other animal, and have it freshly slaughtered to their specifications. Close to eighty viveros operate in NYC, mostly in Northern Manhattan, Brooklyn, Queens, and the Bronx. An outbreak of *Salmonella Haardt* occurred in 2003–2004 that was believed to have originated at a vivero. Community, cultural, and religious practices require access to meat processed in this manner. We arranged to ship Mr. Santiago's specimens to the CDC lab to test for leptospirosis.

Leptospirosis is a reportable disease in New York and all cases get investigated. In the previous decade and a half, there had been thirty-eight cases of human leptospirosis in the city. Most cases occur in returning foreign travelers, but a few locally acquired cases occur just about every year and in all parts of the city. No outbreaks or links among the cases had ever been found. By itself, one possible case of leptospirosis wasn't news, but there was an urgency. Since the patient worked at a live animal market there was a potential risk to other workers. Additionally, the patient's wife and brothers had told doctors at the hospital that he wasn't the first person to get sick. Another worker had taken ill a few weeks earlier. That man reportedly died. Family members did not know the man's name and Mr. Santiago was far too ill to be questioned. Mr. Santiago's brother had additional information. He believed that the man was in his 30s and had gone to a local Bronx hospital in the last two weeks.

The same week the suspect leptospirosis case was reported, and for the next several months, the D❂Ds were consumed with an outbreak of novel influenza type H7N2 among cats housed in a city-run shelter. Most staff, including Veterinary Epidemiologist Sally Slavinski, were busy identifying where the cats had been and who had encountered them. A clinic was also being stood up to test workers.

It is not uncommon for information to reach the health department that turns out not to be true. Often these calls were about suspected meningitis that turned out to be something else of no public health concern. Part of our job is due diligence. With the name of the vivero, I began chasing the rumor of the previous ill worker. I called the vivero but got no answer. We work closely with the OCME, and I reasoned if a young man died under the circumstances described it would be referred to them for investigation. I gave them all the information I had and asked them to check on recent Bronx deaths in young males. My next call was to a colleague in OVS. Deaths need to be reported and are entered into an electronic database. We'd been collaborating with OVS on an automated system to scan death certificates for unusual deaths that might be infectious and for clusters. There are close to 1,000 deaths per week in NYC. Narrowing the age range and geography would reduce the number, but not to something manageable.

I mapped the vivero. The closest hospital was Bronx Lebanon. I trained with the head of the emergency department there, so I called him. He could not recall a young male dying in the emergency department (ED) in the past several weeks suspicious for leptospirosis, or otherwise. Without the decedent's name, all they could do was try to canvas all the staff, an arduous task for a busy ED.

I got a break when I called back the vivero and someone answered. The owner was out of the country, but I reached a supervisor. He confirmed that there was a worker who they had hired recently to help with the seasonal increase in business. He didn't know much about the man and said he hadn't worked in several weeks.

"Did he get sick and die?" I asked.

He put down the phone to confer with staff. I could hear water splashing in the background among the cacophony of animal sounds. When he returned, he confirmed that the worker had died.

"He died from a broken heart," he said.

"What?"

I was told that the worker was to get married, and his fiancée broke it off. He allegedly died shortly after being jilted. They only knew his first name, Omar, and that he might have been from Africa or Jamaica. They didn't know where he lived, if he had any relatives, or any other useful information.

"What about payroll or HR records?" I asked. That got me nowhere. He was paid in cash, off the books.

"What work did he do?"

I was told he did cleanup and that he didn't work with chickens.

I called back Wenhui Liu of OVS and asked him to scan the system for deaths in a person named Omar going back a month, anywhere in the city. About an hour later, Wenhui called me back. He found thirty-four deaths in people with the name Omar, who died in 2016. One person fit the limited description I had given him. Omar Diallo died in the Bronx on December 5. I dialed Dr. Melissa Pasquale at the OCME. Her husband, Dr. Tim Styles, did a public health residency elective with me in 2006 and years later joined the health department in the hospital preparedness program. Melissa found Diallo's file and summarized the investigator's notes.

Bronx Lebanon Hospital had reported the death of a previously well, thirty-seven-year-old African American male who came to the ED by ambulance at 2:30 a.m. on December 5. He complained of body aches and fatigue. He was breathing fast, low on oxygen, and coughing blood. There was no obvious trauma. A radiograph of his lungs was consistent with pneumonia, excess fluid or blood. Laboratory tests showed him to be seriously ill, with blood acidosis and low platelets. His kidneys were also failing. Omar denied recent travel but did have contact with relatives who had recently traveled to Africa. Despite efforts to resuscitate him, he died two hours later.

The OCME is fastidious when completing its task of determining the cause of death in cases that fall under its jurisdiction. These include any deaths where a crime is suspected, suicide, accidents, drug overdoses, sudden deaths in otherwise well persons, deaths that occur while incarcerated, worksite deaths, pregnancy-associated deaths, unattended deaths (such as individuals found dead in their apartments), and deaths that occur under suspicious or unusual circumstances. This case fit their criteria, but Omar's family objected to an autopsy on religious grounds. Objections to autopsy occur and can be overridden, but in this case, because no crime was suspected, no autopsy was performed.

As a result, the medical examiner assigned to the case performed a visual inspection. Other than a few scars on his arms and legs, there was nothing visual that explained his death. The family also refused to allow any blood to be taken, but the OCME had located, retrieved, and stored blood samples taken at the hospital. We arranged to ship those specimens to the CDC's lab for testing.

Leptospirosis has been a concern for NYC dog owners. Anywhere from ten to twenty canine cases occur every year, but this may be an undercount of the true burden as many don't get diagnosed or reported. The disease causes symptoms similar to that in humans and can be fatal. Most cases occur in Brooklyn and Manhattan, and there hasn't been any known transmission from dogs to humans. It is believed that most of the affected dogs were exposed to rodents, specifically rats, or standing water containing rodent urine.

The health department maintains a list of rat reservoirs and known locations of infestations. When we shared the Bronx vivero location with Environmental Health Service (EHS) colleagues they knew the area as a rat reservoir. The vivero was located on a historic Bronx boulevard in a two-story building nestled between a vacant lot and a furniture warehouse. D✪D Marc Paladini accompanied an inspector from EHS to the site. Two cinder block staircases led to the vivero entryway. Immediately to the right of the entry hall was a pen for livestock, mostly goats and sheep, but there were several cows, all packed close together with barely enough room to turn around. On the left were stacked dozens of cages filled with chickens. At the front, near the windows, were poultry display cases. The back of the store held the kill and processing rooms. There were stations for bleeding, steaming, feather removal, and gutting. Between the killing room and a display case with eggs was a narrow room storing trash and an offal counter.

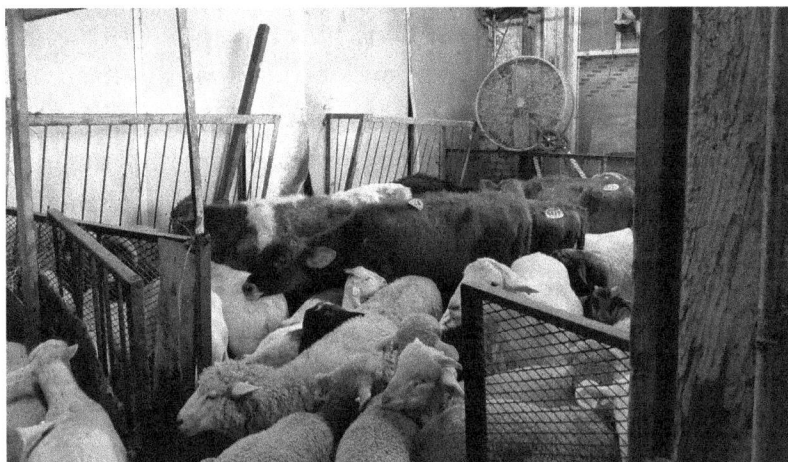

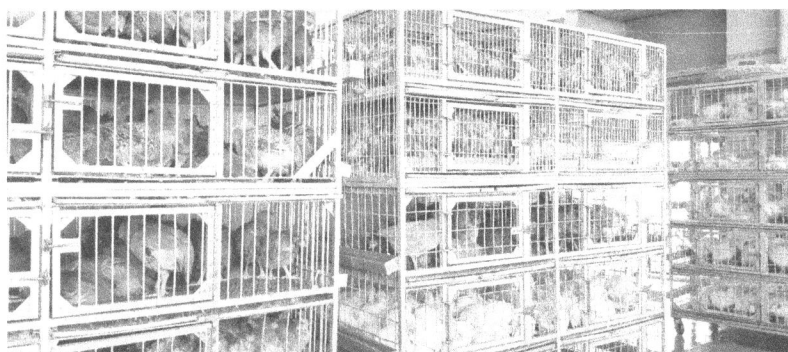

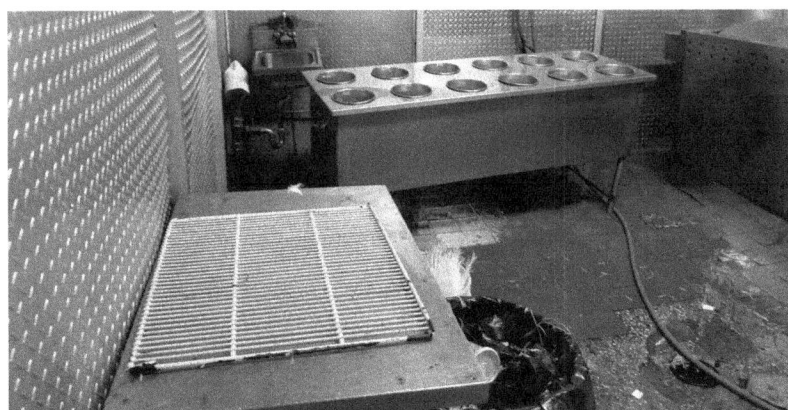

Images from site visit to the vivero–photographs by Marc Paladini

The vivero employed six staff. All were wearing boots, smocks, and heavy-duty gloves at the time of Marc's visit. But no one wore eye protection or face masks. Periodically throughout the day, the work areas were swept and sprayed down with water from a hose. Before going home for the day, bleach is sprayed and left overnight. Marc and the inspector found garbage, construction clutter, as well as rat burrow openings in the sidewalks, building foundation, and ceilings, in addition to copious, fresh rat droppings. The owner was cited and given five days to initiate cleanup before a re-inspection would occur.

Leptospira are bacteria, specifically categorized as spirochetes, like the organism that causes syphilis. As such they don't grow well on artificial media like most bacteria. Diagnosis relies on detecting specific DNA sequences using PCR or through detecting antibodies. There are two species, and many subspecies called serovars. *Leptospira interrogans* is the species that causes disease. *Leptospira* are zoonotic, meaning they circulate in the animal world and humans get exposed by contact with animals or their excreta. Specific *Leptospira* serovars have adapted to a variety of animal hosts which then serve as reservoirs for ongoing transmission. This relationship allows the animals to function as amplifiers—meaning, animals survive infection while excreting large quantities of the bacteria into the environment. While *Leptospira* can be found in hundreds of animal species, only mammals appear to be able to transmit the disease to humans mostly through contact with infected urine. That contact can be through open skin, like cuts and abrasions; through mucous membranes, such as the eyes and mouth; the lungs; or perhaps through ingestion. Infections are associated with exposure to water and outbreaks have occurred during rainy seasons and floods. Most cases occur in tropical climates, particularly in Southeast Asia. *Leptospira* are motile, which may facilitate their entry into cells and organs.

Most cases of leptospirosis are mild. What's more, combined with the diagnostic difficulties it's often misdiagnosed. How sick a person gets depends in part on the person's immune system, health status, as well as the quantity of bacteria, and the strain. Symptoms typically appear one to two weeks after the exposure. The illness begins with fever, which can be as high as 104°F, along with headache, chills, and muscle aches—not all that different from the flu. Red eyes can occur, and the illness can be as short as a few days or as long as several weeks.

The most severe form of leptospirosis is known as Weil's disease and was so named in 1886 by Heidelberg physician, Adolph Weil. He described four patients with fever, jaundice, and kidney and central nervous system involvement. However, it was not until 1915 that Japanese researchers successfully identified the spirochete bacteria by infecting guinea pigs with blood from a patient with Weil's disease. The guinea pigs developed symptoms analogous to human disease and the organism was found in their livers. Weil's disease features kidney and liver failure that leads to jaundice, accumulation of toxic waste products in the blood, and decreased urine production. Platelet counts plummet leading to vascular instability and hemorrhagic complications, which can include the lungs. Meningitis can be a complication, and death due to cardiovascular collapse occurs in 5–15% of patients.

Both Santiago and Diallo had symptoms that fit with Weil's disease and the diagnosis for both was confirmed by the CDC just before New Year's Eve 2016. A review of other staff at the vivero did not uncover any current or past illness suspicious for leptospirosis. We took it a step further and re-interviewed all reported leptospirosis cases going back six months. Of the six cases, three reported international travel, to Costa Rica, Thailand,

and multiple countries in Southeast Asia. However, none of the six had visited the vivero.

Once Mr. Santiago recovered, he was interviewed with the aid of an interpreter, DOD Elrinda Amoroso. He was new to the vivero and worked six days a week beginning the Monday after Thanksgiving until he became ill. The workdays of Mr. Santiago and Mr. Diallo overlapped on November 28–30. The last time Mr. Santiago saw Mr. Diallo he said the latter seemed unwell. Mr. Santiago reported frequently seeing rats around the vivero, but never came in direct contact with them. He only worked with poultry and performed all jobs including killing, feather removal, processing, and equipment cleaning. He was also responsible for cleaning the animal pens, and he did this without gloves or a mask. On breaks, he and others often would eat over the sink in the prep room. Mr. Santiago said he often got cuts on his arms and hands, and that he did not always wear gloves. He confirmed that no respiratory protection was used. Mr. Diallo worked in the kill room and was responsible for killing chickens, using the steam device to loosen feathers, and cleaning up. He reportedly did not work with animals other than chickens.

How had the two men become infected? While leptospirosis can infect ruminants, like cows and goats, it is more commonly linked to rodents. It is unlikely that either had come in direct contact with rats. But for certain there was rat urine and feces in and around the vivero, and it seems likely that water from the high-pressure hose could have aerosolized rat urine which then could have infected the men through either the respiratory, mucous membrane, or open wound routes. The vivero was instructed to provide workers with respiratory and eye protection. In addition to always wearing gloves and smocks, workers were to take steps to minimize animal scraps that were food for rats and secure the trash. The vivero was also directed to contract with an exterminator and immediately contact the health department should they learn of illness in any worker or patron.

We checked in with the vivero right after the new year to make sure all workers were well by phone, and Marc along, with Gili, another D✪D who was a native Spanish speaker, visited again in early February. All seemed back to normal, meaning chickens were still losing their heads and rats were still running around, but there had been no new human illnesses. We had also communicated to area hospitals to be on alert for patients presenting with symptoms compatible with leptospirosis who reported exposure to rodents. We didn't get any calls. A plan to trap and test rats was formulated, though it would take weeks to put in place, and much longer to get the results.

Leptospirosis, often called a neglected tropical disease, burst onto the international stage in 2000 when participants in the Eco-Challenge-Sabah returned to their home countries and took ill.[106] The multi-sport endurance race held in Malaysia Borneo, featured legs of jungle trekking, swimming, kayaking, climbing, cycling, and spelunking. Over 300 athletes from twenty-seven countries participated. Of those that CDC investigators were able to reach, eighty had the symptoms of leptospirosis, twenty-nine required hospitalization, and 68% of those tested were positive. Swallowing or exposure to river water was the suspected source and all participants recovered.

Five years later, and closer to home, a case of leptospirosis in a New York State resident exposed an outbreak among participants of an endurance swamp race held near Tampa, Florida.[107] Forty-four racers had leptospirosis symptoms and 45% of persons tested were positive. Most participants incurred cuts and abrasions to their legs from the sharp-edged swamp foliage, which may have been the entry point for the *Leptospira*. If global warming results in more of the Earth being covered by water, we can expect an increased risk for leptospirosis.

Just blocks north of the vivero, on that major Bronx thoroughfare, there are apartment buildings built in the early twentieth century. The neighborhood features landmarks such as the Bronx County Courthouse and Yankee Stadium. My paternal grandparents lived in one of those apartment buildings at 161st Street and I have memories of the art deco building lobby and crossing the street to the park and stadium. Those memories came flooding back when on February 9, 2017, we received another leptospirosis case report. The man lived in a basement apartment and had been hospitalized for six days with a flu-like illness that included liver and kidney failure. The hospital had sent a specimen to a commercial lab who reported the leptospirosis result to the department. We sent specimens to the CDC, and they confirmed the diagnosis. The man didn't work but reported doing cleaning in the building which had a problem with rats. He had not made any visits to the vivero, which stood a mere 500 feet away.

Staff from the Departments of Health and Buildings descended on the dwelling on February 13 to inspect. A rat was seen in the kitchen of a basement apartment, and fresh rat droppings, along with accessible food scraps, were found in the trash compactor rooms in each building wing. Twelve active rat burrows were found and abundant debris suitable for nesting material was found in the courtyard. The next day, the basement apartments were evacuated and padlocked.

I attended the community meeting the night of February 15 in case there were any questions about the investigation or leptospirosis that NYC Health Commissioner Bassett couldn't answer. The meeting was held in the building's lobby, a space about the size of a handball court with mirrored pillars and hallways extending to the left and right. There weren't enough chairs, so many stood, making the scene more like a crowd anxious for a store to open on Black Friday. Tenants packed closer to the door, while Dr. Bassett and NYC officials were by the elevators. Reporters with cameras, some using their phones, waited to ask their questions. The space was packed and warm. Many department and agency representatives wore jackets with their division names on them. I did not. It was evident from the outset that the tenants were not interested in explanations or a treatise on leptospirosis. They had grievances. Many were in legal battles with the landlord over delayed repairs and were reluctant to allow repairs for fear that the cost would fall on them, or their lawsuits would be rendered moot.

Dr. Bassett wasn't at her best, and I felt the message was off topic. We needed to lay out an immediate action plan, using all available resources. Instead, the message was imprecise about what would happen and when it would occur. Dr. Bassett remained calm, but the crowd spoke over one another, with an occasional raised voice. Public Advocate Letitia James tried to give the residents practical action steps, but few were able to hear her. As soon as the meeting ended, I scurried out and down the block to the subway to head home, thinking along the way how the risk for additional cases was low but fixing the rat problem, not just in this building, but throughout the neighborhood and city, was a monumental task.

Rat ecology follows the laws of nature. In times of limited habitat and food, reproduction rates are low. If there's ample food as there is in NYC, rats can reproduce quickly. The gestation period for the brown rat, *Rattus norvegicus*, is about three weeks and litters can be as large as twelve pups. Poisoning rats is a short-term solution. Some rats die, but that means there is more food available, so the reproductive rate goes up. As a result, the population quickly recovers. Another plan getting traction is to feed rats food laced with contraceptives. A small pilot program in a NYC park gave up on the idea after a few months as there was way too much non-laced food for rats to eat. The solution is to eliminate their food source and habitat. Every garbage receptacle, be it in an apartment, basement compactor room, street corner, or alley behind a restaurant needs to be rat impenetrable. The city is moving in this direction with new legislation requiring trash receptacles to be animal impenetrable. As daunting as this task sounds, eliminating rat habitats is practically impossible. Rats can burrow in parks, gnaw through structures, and even live in trees. The trapping at the vivero and surrounding areas found that of fifty rats tested, twenty-six were positive for leptospirosis. The best plan to prevent human and canine leptospirosis is to take rats off the NYC meal plan.

CHAPTER 14

It Was Only a Question of When

My first public health job was in a Midwest city from 1996–1999. It was a tumultuous three years in which the health commissioner changed twice, and the department was marred by scandals. The experience inspired me to write the novel, *The Rat Catcher and the Mole*. One common refrain from epidemiologists of that era was that another influenza pandemic was only a matter of time. In the twentieth century, there had been three influenza pandemics and one scare. In the late 1990s, we were said to be "due" for another pandemic. Underlying that prediction were the nature of the influenza virus and the ease of humans to travel great distances. As most people know, influenza infects a wide array of species, not just humans. With waterfowl and swine serving as mixing vessels, and influenza's predilection to mutate, it was like rolling dice, and epidemiologists believed that eventually the dice would land with snake eyes.

It had been thirty years since the last pandemic. The CDC, along with state and local health departments, were anxious and crafting response plans. All this changed in 2002 when SARS, a non-influenza zoonotic virus emerged, circled the globe, and caused a relatively constrained pandemic. SARS put humanity on notice that influenza wasn't the only threat. With human incursions into previously undisturbed ecosystems, we were opening the proverbial Pandora's box of viruses. The next coronavirus to emerge did so in 2012. MERS-CoV didn't spawn a pandemic, but it exceeded its predecessor with 35% mortality. Seven years later, a novel H1N1 influenza virus emerged and caused another pandemic. It is true now as it was then that it is only a matter of time until the next pandemic.

During the COVID-19 pandemic, I created log files, something I was in the habit of doing for large outbreaks so that I wouldn't forget the details that often don't make it into official reports. The COVID-19 files contain emails, text messages, meeting notes, conversation highlights, charts, graphs, data analyses, links to media stories, and journal article summaries, as well as my thoughts, frustrations, and protests. The twenty-seven files cover the first twenty-nine months of the pandemic. The files contain over 4,200 pages and more than a million words. Summarizing it all in a chapter is a task nearly as insurmountable as the pandemic, and though cliché, the volume of material could fill a book or two. I did try to capture all that transpired, but when the draft chapter length exceeded 20,000 words, and I had only reached midway in the second wave, I reconsidered the approach. Many themes emerged during the pandemic, but the one that stood out above all the others was the politicization of public health. If you want to know all the gritty details of what really happened behind the walls of government, you'll just have to wait for the next book.

After the attacks of 9/11, and before the anthrax letters, then NYC Health Commissioner Neal Cohen invited several Disease Control staff to his office to discuss the situation. I attended but was the most junior of the invited staff. Commissioner Cohen was a psychiatrist and recognized that he wasn't well-positioned to make decisions about infectious diseases or bioterrorism, so he placed great trust in his staff who were. During the COVID-19 pandemic, I often thought about those days, and while they were incredibly arduous and stressful, we knew that our leaders had our backs. We knew that we would be listened to and that decisions would follow not just science, but common sense, and not be motivated by political expediency and aspirational agendas.

To understand the environment in which the department found itself in 2020–2022, we must revisit an outbreak that happened five years earlier. As detailed in Chapter 12, an outbreak of Legionnaires' disease occurred in the South Bronx in the summer of 2015. Within a day of beginning the outbreak investigation, the putative source was identified, subsequently proven by state-of-the-art laboratory methods, and remediated. Mayor Bill de Blasio then insisted that our environmental inspectors break into businesses, which legally they could not do, to continue testing every possible source in the Bronx. Dan Kass, who was then the deputy commissioner of the Environmental Health Division, and over the inspection staff, refused on several grounds, including that the effort was a waste of resources for the sole purpose of optics. The health commissioner at the time, Dr. Mary Bassett, was pressured to fire Dan. She also refused. New York City had one of the most respected health departments in the United States, if not the world. In my years with the department, our counsel was sought after by numerous state and city health departments as well as countries across the globe. Both Dan and Mary soon left the department on their own terms, but what remained was de Blasio's animosity and distrust.

Political and public health goals need not be in conflict.

Common ground can be reached that protects the integrity of both yet advances the needs of the population. This occurs through mutual respect, trust, and honest communication. When lives are at stake there is no place for vindictiveness, rather adherence to science and facts is paramount. De Blasio made a brief and utterly unsuccessful run for the Democratic nomination for president in 2020 and toyed with a run for a congressional seat. I like to think that his seeming authoritarianism played a role in his political demise, but it is likely broader than that. As reported by his former press secretary, a woman, in a *New York Times* article, she felt de Blasio's signature move was to, "dig in on an untenable position against the advice of his staff."[108] Other female staffers felt "marginalized" and his "condescension."[109] Twenty-two female City Hall staffers left their posts in the first three years de Blasio was in office. The mayor's management and apparent predilection to mansplain were credited for the departures.[110] What's more, male coworkers were described as adopting his style.

Most health department employees are women, and many during my tenure were in leadership positions. Five of the six assistant commissioners in the Divisions of Disease Control for much of the 2010s were women. All were experienced, competent, trusted, and dedicated public health servants. In my limited, and arm's length observations, de Blasio surrounded himself with young, ambitious, and inexperienced staff, who felt obliged to him and followed his orders without question. They also appeared willing to adopt his predilection to bully.

In the nightmare, I am standing at the railing of a boardwalk, looking over a pristine beach. People sunbathe, frolic in the surf, and play in the sand unaware of the danger. Miles out at sea, a tsunami has formed and is heading toward the shore. The tsunami represents a new, yet anticipated challenge to public health, and is not made of water but of steel in the form of planes and ships. What the vessels carry are part 2002 SARS, part 2009 pandemic influenza, and part LD—a twenty-first-century pandemic strain.

The first rumble began on January 5, 2020, when I read a Yahoo headline and clicked on the link. The story was about an outbreak of pneumonia in China.[111] The mysterious illness had sickened forty-four people in the inland city of Wuhan and eleven were in serious condition. I copied the link and emailed it to several of my fellow D✪Ds. Joel Ackelsberg replied with a link to ProMED posts from a few days earlier reporting that influenza, adenovirus, and other common viruses had been ruled out. A seafood market was implicated. D✪D Scott Harper, the bureau's influenza expert, had been monitoring the posts, and queried his influenza contacts at the CDC, but they knew little more than we did. Everybody immediately thought back to SARS, despite the Chinese government asserting otherwise.

When SARS emerged in 2002, it too, was linked to animal markets in China. The virus was a new, cross-species jump of a zoonotic coronavirus. SARS infected a little over 8,400 people across the globe with approximately 900 deaths. Most patients were exposed in hospitals. We escaped SARS, as no cases occurred in NYC, not that we didn't look for them or have close calls. A NYC businessman traveled to Hong Kong and stayed on the same floor in the hotel where the SARS outbreak began. Had he decided to return home instead of continuing his trip, NYC might have had the outbreak Vietnam experienced.

Dr. Mike Phillips, who was our EIS assignee, attended an infectious disease conference in the city that had many international attendees. One of those, a doctor from Singapore, had cared for a patient with an unknown pneumonia before coming to NYC. The patient had returned from a trip to Hong Kong. The physician became ill but improved enough to travel to NYC. He was diagnosed with atypical pneumonia, and on the flight home was removed in Frankfort, Germany, and placed in isolation. He was diagnosed with SARS as were his wife and mother-in-law who traveled with him. Mike, as was his custom, sat in the back of the conference hall, as did a Singaporean physician.

We watched and read the scant news coming out of China and met to discuss the potential implications. As each day passed since the last case onset of January 5, we cheered no new cases. The Huanan seafood market, where the outbreak is believed to have begun, had been closed. Poultry had been culled. Did this end the outbreak before it had a chance to catch fire? We were optimistic, after all, we had dodged the SARS bullet. Chinese health officials had quickly identified a novel coronavirus and developed a test. The world had little insight as to what was transpiring in Wuhan. Unfortunately, we only got to count eight days before a new case was announced. The new case wasn't in Wuhan though. It was in Thailand. And then a case appeared in Japan. January 13 was the day we officially started preparing for the tsunami.

On January 17, 2020, the CDC distributed a health alert detailing the patient under investigation (PUI) for COVID-19 criteria for public health practitioners to distribute to their medical community:

Patients in the United States who meet the following criteria should be evaluated as a PUI in association with the outbreak of 2019-nCoV in Wuhan City, China.

1) Fever AND symptoms of lower respiratory illness (e.g., cough, shortness of breath)
—and in the last 14 days before symptom onset,

- *History of travel from Wuhan City, China*

–or–

- *Close contact with a person who is under investigation for 2019–nCOV while that person was ill.*

2) Fever OR symptoms of lower respiratory illness (e.g., cough, shortness of breath)
–and in the last 14 days before symptom onset,

- *Close contact with an ill laboratory-confirmed 2019-nCoV patient.[112]*

The CDC created a hotline for state and local health departments to call to report suspected cases and to arrange testing, which was limited due to a shortage of testing supplies. The prevailing theory that the first cases would occur in travelers from Wuhan, China, was based on the belief that severe disease was common and would bring the person to medical attention.

By January 27, there were over 2,800 cases reported in China with eighty-one deaths. The illness had spread beyond Wuhan, China, to Hong Kong, Taiwan, and Macau. Beyond China to Japan, Korea, Singapore, Thailand, Vietnam, and the United States. The first COVID-19 case *diagnosed* in the United States was in a thirty-five-year-old man from Washington State who had traveled to Wuhan, China. He became ill upon his return on January 15 and was diagnosed five days later. Joining the first case in Washington State were cases in California, Chicago, and two in Arizona. New countries were being added to the list almost daily: Canada, France, Australia, Malaysia, and Nepal came next. In the meantime, we'd been slowly preparing—designing forms and updating databases.

The CDC was screening arriving passengers from Wuhan,

China, but many arrived well in NYC and then became ill. We'd been receiving calls from NYC medical providers seeing ill patients with recent travel. We investigated them but none met the CDC criteria. They either weren't sick enough or had another diagnosis, like influenza. The Mayor's Office asked why we didn't have any cases here. The implication being that we weren't doing our jobs. It was almost as if we had to compete with LA and Chicago who had cases. We followed the CDC rules, but not without trepidation. We knew based on the limited news and natural history of viral respiratory infections that the majority of COVID-19 illnesses were mild. The overwhelming probability favored mild cases arriving in NYC, but our hands felt tied. We discussed testing mild disease, some of us arguing in favor, but we were voted down, and we stuck to CDC's criteria.

It didn't take long before City Hall was in our faces. A deputy mayor demanded to see our doctor-of-the-week (DOW) protocol, an innocuous document that detailed the responsibilities of the medical epidemiologist rotation. Each week a physician, or senior level epidemiologist, served as the DOW to handle incoming calls, questions, or reports that were other than routine. The protocol had little to do with COVID-19. It was likely some constituents had complained to the mayor that they were refused testing because they didn't meet CDC criteria. Newly minted deputy commissioner, and soon-to-be COVID-19 incident commander, Dr. Demetre Daskalakis showed the DOW protocol document to the deputy mayor, and we heard no more about it. But the damage was done, it signaled that the mayor did not trust the DODs to do his bidding and it was a warning shot across the bow. The very next day, ICS was activated.

After 9/11, Rick Heffernan, Farzad Mostashari, Debjani Das, and myself, along with others, developed the emergency department syndromic surveillance system. Syndromic surveillance is an ancillary surveillance system to monitor disease in a population before a diagnosis is made. It is rooted in the theory that should an event happen, be it a natural pandemic or bioterrorism attack, people will present to area EDs in sufficient numbers with similar symptoms as to "signal" public health authorities that there's a problem. The NYC syndromic surveillance system expanded and evolved over the twenty-plus years I oversaw the program, and it had proved valuable in many ways other than its original intent. For years, we used it to monitor influenza activity and severity. We now tuned it to detect COVID-19. The problem we immediately faced though was that it was influenza season and many of the symptoms overlapped, but if COVID-19 took off we expected to see a rise in ED visits. The Chinese CDC posted on their website an epidemic curve. It was as steep as any I had ever seen.

Marie, the public health nurse on phone duty, forwarded me a call on January 29 from a surgeon in charge of ECMO at a Brooklyn hospital. ECMO stands for extracorporeal membrane oxygenation and it's a machine used to temporarily function as a person's lungs. Blood is removed from the body, pumped through a machine that adds oxygen and removes carbon dioxide, and then returns the blood to the body. As you can surmise, this process is fraught with potential complications. Only people deathly ill get placed on ECMO. The patient was in his late forties, and had hypertension and type 2 diabetes, but otherwise had been well. His illness began with a cough, and he presented to a local hospital where he rapidly decompensated, requiring transfer for advanced medical care. The patient wasn't getting enough oxygen, and the chest radiograph showed disease throughout both lungs. Tests for influenza and RSV were negative. He worked as a ride-share driver and reported frequent trips to JFK International Airport to pick up fares. As I heard the details of the laboratory and clinical findings, I became convinced that he had COVID-19. It seemed inconceivable to me that in a city with business connections to the parts of the world where COVID-19 was raging and frequent international travel, that we wouldn't have a case four weeks into the pandemic. We were following, to the letter, the CDC's recommendations on who to send for testing. If you hadn't traveled from an area with cases and didn't have lower airway disease or had been exposed to a known case, we weren't allowed to test you as resources were still tight.

Former D❂D Dr. Sharon Balter, who now worked in LA, told us she was sending specimens to the CDC that didn't strictly meet the criteria. I suspected other jurisdictions were doing the same, but we stubbornly held back. Incredibly shortsighted, I argued on more than one occasion, including the team meeting I called to discuss the ride-share driver's illness. With most of the D❂D COVID-19 council squeezed into Marci's office, I presented the case, highlighting the similarities the patient had to the case reports coming out of China and elsewhere. Although the patient didn't himself travel, he had exposure to travelers. At the time, masks were not yet recommended, and the CDC did not believe the virus was airborne. I was voted down, and the patient wasn't tested, well, not until several months later. I advised the physicians caring for the patient to collect and freeze specimens, as at some point, we'd circle back and test them. I then directed them to use COVID-19 infection control precautions.

Many immigrant communities in NYC don't trust the government and this wariness extends to the medical profession. I knew there was much commerce, both legal and illegal, with China—people flying back and forth and a brisk black-market trade. I worried that returning travelers or their household contacts who became ill might not seek healthcare, or at least not mainstream healthcare, that would bring them to our attention. I imagined a scenario in which COVID-19 cases were occurring in an insulated community in NYC. Worst-case scenario would be mildly ill people who wouldn't seek health care or if they did, their providers wouldn't inform us out of ignorance or fear. I urged ICS to do more outreach to the Chinese medical community. The true nature of COVID-19 disease is mild illness, that is until it finds an immune vulnerable host with pre-existing health conditions. I worried that we'd miss the opportunity to prevent an onslaught. I also suspected that the first case or cases might not have traveled to Wuhan or even be connected to the Chinese community. As we moved through the first weeks of February, we fielded numerous calls, but no patient met the testing criteria. In a little more than a month, the global pandemic had outpaced MERS and exceeded the total number of SARS cases in 2003–2004. Yet, the number of US cases was less than ten. The numbers didn't seem believable.

During Ebola, although we had just the one case, we traced his every step in the days before onset to ensure we were aware of any potential exposures. Ebola, though deadlier, was less worrisome than COVID-19 because it is not transmitted by the respiratory route nor before symptom onset. COVID-19 possesses both features. Contact tracing was never something we believed could be done during a viral pandemic and it wasn't a part of the pandemic influenza plan. For a respiratory virus, transmitted rapidly and efficiently by mildly ill or asymptomatic persons, we didn't believe in its public health value. Contacting thousands of new cases each day to elicit contacts, and then monitoring them and their contacts for weeks to ensure compliance with isolation and quarantine was deemed impractical in a Democratic society. Especially one as divided as the United States, with huge swaths of anti-government factions. We didn't think many people would answer their phones and if they did, they would be reluctant to disclose their contacts. Pandemic modelers believed that we had only three days to identify, interview the case, solicit their close contacts, locate and speak with the contacts, and implement control measures.

One of the topics that routinely surfaces during disease outbreaks is patient confidentiality. ICS took up this issue, though it was one the bureaus in our division had long resolved. We expected that the media would hound governmental officials for information about the first COVID-19 patients discovered in NYC but once cases were too numerous to count, they'd move on to other topics. Our duty as public health practitioners is to preserve patient confidentiality. Even minimal demographic data, such as age, sex, and borough, can allow a determined investigative reporter to identify a patient. When our public information officer confessed ignorance of our confidentiality policy, we had reasons to be concerned. That same afternoon, the CDC announced that person-to-person COVID-19 transmission had been documented in Chicago and the WHO declared COVID-19 a global health emergency. However, it was still relatively calm in the office. People pondered the recent illnesses that circulated in our office in the past month. People had brief flu-like illnesses, followed by a persistent cough with copious mucus. Maybe COVID-19 was already here, meaning right **here**!

It was just after 5:00 p.m. on January 30, and I was preparing for my bike ride home. I suspected that a nine-hour workday would soon be a rare luxury. Demetre and Marci came down the hallway and stopped in front of my cubicle. Demetre did the talking, saying he thinks we need new classifications. CDC was using person under investigation (PUI) to indicate a person with illness and risk factors meeting COVID-19 testing criteria. We adopted the same designation for consistency, but Demetre thought that we needed a different designation, one he called a pre-PUI (PPUI).

"Puppy?" I replied.

Demetre explained that when we designate a patient as a PUI, city hall gets anxious and starts bugging him. If we reclassify as a PPUI, we won't have to tell City Hall. We can therefore avoid their prying eyes looking over our shoulders. While I appreciated not having City Hall micromanaging us, I couldn't endorse the Wile E. Coyote idea.

"We're going to have cases," I told Demetre. "Of this there is no doubt. Better to get it over with sooner than later."

My bike ride home from our office in Long Island City, Queens, takes about thirty minutes. It was a time to decompress and process the events of the day. I thought about Demetre's words. Like Wile E. Coyote, with the Road Runner, and Daffy Duck, with Bugs Bunny, he was conniving to outwit City Hall. At the time I didn't see City Hall as the obstacle, at least not the most critical one. By following the CDC's strict criteria for testing we were missing cases. If we took too long and missed too many cases, the pandemic would appear to have arrived out of nowhere. While that would undoubtedly freak out City Hall, it would make containment that much more impossible. When I got home, I sent an email to the Surveillance and Epidemiology Branch leadership urging us to modify our interpretation of the CDC testing criteria. Since mild disease was more common and travel to Wuhan had been suspended for the past two weeks, we needed to go off the CDC script. Test people who had COVID-19 symptoms and more nuanced risk factors, not requiring lower respiratory tract disease—such as public-facing professions, like airport workers, baristas, and ride-share drivers.

My anxiety about missing cases only grew as we watched the outbreak spread throughout China and the planet. There were cases in over twenty countries, so any foreign travel could be a risk. To make matters worse, testing supplies were still a limited and precious resource. The CDC lab was preparing test kits to send to state laboratories, but it couldn't happen fast enough, and when they finally shipped there was a problem with one of the reagents. Meanwhile, commercial labs were working on developing their assays and having them approved by the FDA. It was a horrible place to be, wedged between the suspicion of cases and the inability to test them. And did we really have any hope of preventing transmission in NYC?

The end of January arrived with no good news. COVID-19 case counts in China topped 10,000. The sixth US case, a Chicago man, was the husband of a traveler to China. A letter to the editor appeared in *The New England Journal of Medicine* that reported a COVID-19 case in a person who was exposed to a person before symptom onset. The German citizen met with the businesswoman on January 20 and 21 in Munich. He developed a sore throat, fever, and muscle aches on January 24 which resolved two days later, and he went back to work on January 27. The asymptomatic woman, who was from Shanghai, became ill on the plane back to China where she subsequently tested positive. Contact tracing at the Munich office identified three more COVID-19 cases, all of which were mild.[113]

The dreaded scenario for infectious disease control is a disease transmitted by the respiratory route, with a short incubation period, that is transmissible one or more days before symptoms appear. The incubation period in the German case was three or four days, and one of the secondary cases had no contact with the Chinese businesswoman, meaning transmission was from the coworker. If a person with COVID-19 is contagious two days before they show symptoms and it only takes three days to get sick, that leaves public health officials limited time for the initial sick person to get tested, return the laboratory results, perform a contact investigation, locate, speak with, and employ quarantine measures to the contacts. Multiply the task 10,000-fold and you get the idea of the daunting task the COVID-19 pandemic presented.

The CDC eventually revised the PUI criteria, amending the travel requirement to anywhere in China, but retained the severe illness criterion. It was four weeks into the pandemic, and we still hadn't identified a COVID-19 case in NYC and the email to my colleagues imploring that we veer from CDC's rigidity received zero response. I sensed that my colleagues knew we were likely missing detecting community transmission, but we stuck with CDC's criteria and waited for PHL to have the ability to test. Additional news came from the CDC. The 195 diplomats who evacuated from Wuhan were placed under a federal fourteen-day quarantine order on a California military base. It was the first time in fifty years that such an order had been issued. The order was issued because a person attempted to exit voluntary quarantine. What about all the domestic travelers who have returned from China? If we were to follow the CDC's lead, every returning traveler from China, not yet fourteen days past arrival, should be issued an order to quarantine.

On Friday, January 31, we had a conference call with public health officials from California. They reported having tested sixty people, many of whom did not meet the PUI criteria, and we hadn't requested testing on a single patient. Not that we weren't getting calls and requests. That same day, we got a call about a sixty-two-year-old man who returned from China, became ill seven days later, never sought care, recovered, and was told—presumably by the CDC—that he had been exposed to a case while on the plane. We also received word from a college student health center about a student from Wuhan with a sore throat, cough, and runny nose, but no fever. The student lived with four roommates, thankfully off campus, and had isolated. We didn't ask the CDC to test.

The next day, Saturday, February 1, I was at my desk in a cold, empty office. An article appeared in *The Wall Street Journal* claiming that the United States had declared a public health emergency and that all returning travelers from China were subject to a fourteen-day quarantine. However, the orders didn't come from the CDC. They were issued by the federal government, another salvo against public health.

The night before, a twenty-seven-year-old woman showed up in an ED having returned from China. She had a cough and fever and just before discharge became short of breath. Our first PUI. During the morning's ICS meeting, I listened to an hour of a planning discussion on setting up quarantine hotels. By all accounts, when community transmission of COVID-19 takes off, it is going to be big—bigger than all the hotel rooms in the city. Puzzled, I asked why people can't quarantine at home. Demetre, the incident commander, stated that it was the commissioner of health's decision, which I highly doubted—it was more likely the order came from City Hall. In an attempt to inject humor into the dire situation, Demetre quipped that we'd been given lemons, and we were going to make lemonade. I didn't find it funny and was angry that public health policy was being crafted by politicians. The plan was shortsighted, and I wanted to at least have a discussion and propose alternatives to the commissioner. I was shut down. I responded to Demetre, and all the ICS staff in the room and on the call that we weren't making lemonade, "We're making urine." The comment set Demetre off. He went on a several-minute tirade, the gist was that if any other person were serving as incident commander I would be beheaded. At the break, I pulled Marci aside and asked if I should leave the meeting. I didn't wait for her answer as she walked off to speak with Demetre. I headed back to my cubicle to construct a surveillance plan.

Fourteen days is a long time to be stuck in a hotel, even for a tourist able to take in the sights, let alone a person in isolation or quarantine. During the early 1990s, I worked as a pediatrician treating homeless kids living in City-run shelters. Many of the families were housed in hotels that otherwise couldn't fill their vacancies. These hotels were not luxury by any stretch of the imagination and were usually near airports or in parts of the city with few services or access to transportation. Persons placed in a hotel would need supplies, medical care, and emotional support. Fourteen days of quarantine, as we learned during the Ebola case, is difficult to endure and compliance would be much greater if our plan allowed people to stay in their homes. We needed to reconsider this wayward and unsustainable path.

I viewed the plan to use hotels to house people under quarantine as an "optical delusion." A way for the mayor to show the governor, with whom he would engage in an epic pissing match, the public, and other cities, that he was in charge and standing bravely before the oncoming tsunami. I didn't realize it at the time, but over the course of the next two years it became clear that politicians, despite the evidence before their eyes, believed they could dictate the path of the pandemic. I admit that the hotels served a purpose for isolation and quarantine as some people either had no place to stay or preferred to remain away from family members, but they played a very minor role during the pandemic. As the pandemic waves arrived, hotel quarantine became unsustainable, and the overwhelming majority of cases and contacts were quarantined in their homes.

The first NYC PUI tested negative. We'd have a handful more PUIs in February as we awaited testing to be ready at the PHL and the Wadsworth State Laboratory. A one-year-old with a fever and cough had been in China. The influenza test was negative. The D⊗D investigating the patient was becoming anxious and wanted to declare the child a PUI and arrange for testing. But something about the patient struck me as odd. I reviewed her past medical record and noted that she had reasons to suspect an alternate diagnosis. I asked the hospital to test for RSV, a common virus in this age group that causes similar symptoms. RSV was positive. Crisis postponed.

The case count in China vaulted past 30,000. Li Wenliang, the Wuhan Chinese physician who warned the country on social media about the virus, and endured reprimand by the government, died from COVID-19. If there wasn't already high anxiety among healthcare workers, the news was hardly reassuring. There were burgeoning outbreaks in several countries, most notably Iran and Italy, making airport screening more complicated. Japan announced the quarantine of 3,700 people on a cruise ship after a case was identified on board and it wasn't too long after that we learned there were over sixty cases onboard. Yet in the United States, there were still just twelve known cases, and fewer than 300 had been approved for testing.

I decided to spend my time working on a surveillance system to determine whether the virus was in NYC. The idea was to identify mildly ill patients who made an ED visit and tested negative for influenza. If we acted quickly enough, we could collect the negative influenza test swabs before they were disposed of, ship them to the CDC, and have them tested for SARS-CoV-2. We'd pick ED locations that represented different parts of the city, it was something we'd done before, it's called sentinel surveillance. Chicago and LA came up with the same idea and the CDC agreed to perform the testing and coordinate the effort. I drafted the plan and sent it up the ICS chain at the end of the first week of February. Our successes during emergencies are in large part because we are committed to overcoming any and all obstacles, a credit to our collective resourcefulness and perseverance. What wasn't yet obvious was how deeply and repeatedly our resourcefulness and perseverance would be tested, not just with the sentinel plan, but throughout the pandemic response.

The weekly ED syndromic surveillance numbers for influenza-like illness (ILI) began to trend up, but was it due to influenza or COVID-19? Rob Mathes, the lead syndromic surveillance analyst, devised a way to tell. We compared positive influenza tests to ED ILI visits over time. The numbers wouldn't match because more people get tested for influenza than visit EDs for ILL, but we believed that the ratio and trend would be informative. If the gap between positive tests and visits closed or the lines crossed to show more visits than tests, that might indicate that COVID-19 was circulating. Later improvements would allow us to track the proportion of ED visits for ILI that tested positive for influenza, but by that time we had SARS-CoV-2 test results to monitor. However, the first look was somewhat reassuring. As ILI increased so did the positive influenza laboratory tests.

The week of February 11 was my week to be the SurvEpi branch director. The COVID-19 case count in China had exceeded 40,000. Outside of mainland China, there were less than 400 cases and only twelve confirmed cases were in the United

States. None were in NYC. That's because testing still was only available at the CDC. It felt like we were tourists milling about in a beachfront hotel awaiting evacuation instructions as the tsunami approached. A journal article was shared that reported details about the first COVID-19 patients. All had evidence of pneumonia, two-thirds had exposure to the Huanan seafood market, and one-third required ICU care; 15% of patients died.[114] We also started hearing of cases with gastrointestinal instead of respiratory symptoms, as well as cases in healthcare workers. One case was believed to have infected ten healthcare workers, reminiscent of the 2002 SARS pandemic.

A typical day as SurvEpi branch director entailed a series of conference calls. At 9:00 a.m. was the SurvEpi team call, followed at 10:00 by the general ICS call, and then at 11:30 the SurvEpi forward planning team where we attempted to anticipate what data to collect to inform policy decisions that we weren't already collecting. At 1:00, there was a NYS and NYC health departments call, at 2:00 the CDC all-state call, at 3:00 the SurvEpi and lab branches call, followed at 4:00 by the ICS executive committee call. The news of the day was that one of the targets in the CDC's test kit had failed and had to be removed, delaying our ability to test for COVID-19 locally.

The sentinel surveillance proposal to screen people who are negative for influenza was stalled. Demetre and the commissioner postponed deciding for another week. What to bring to City Hall, and when, was plotted to not attract too many questions or concerns. It seemed that Demetre and the commissioner feared how City Hall would react to a positive test. A sticking point was that to avoid having to obtain patient consent, the surveillance design required that specimen collection be anonymous. We wouldn't know patient names and therefore could not implement control measures. It was yet another false concern. By the time the results returned, it would be too late to do any intervention. Recall that persons infected with COVID-19 are believed to be contagious two days before symptoms. With mild symptoms, people likely don't seek medical care for a day or even longer after symptoms begin, waiting to see how the illness progresses. Add in the time to collect, test the specimen for influenza, return a negative, and then gather the specimens to ship to the CDC to perform the COVID-19 test, verify a positive result, and send back results, it would, at minimum, a week, but likely longer, during which time the person was out and about in the community. The name of the person was irrelevant at this point as it would be too late. The optical delusion problem arose again. How would it *look* if the first case diagnosed in NYC was an unnamed person who was neither isolated nor had their contacts identified? The reality was that this had likely already happened. The reason we didn't already know it was because our collective heads, at the direction of the CDC, were buried in the sand.

It was the last weekend of February, and I was on the health department overnight call. There were two physicians on call after hours seven days a week. Some weeks were quiet, others hectic. Fifty countries outside of China had COVID-19 cases and we knew about large outbreaks in Italy, Korea, and Iran. The details of an outbreak at the Washington State long-term care facility were just coming to light and the risk to healthcare workers and the elderly were clearly in focus. It had been nearly two weeks since our last PUI, but no one expected that NYC would escape the pandemic unscathed.

That Saturday at 4:30 p.m., the head of infection control at a local hospital called to discuss two staff members, a married couple, who recently returned from a three-week visit to visit family in a country experiencing a COVID-19 wave. Both were mildly ill, but their symptoms and laboratory tests were consistent with COVID-19. Nasal swabs for testing were being held in the hospital laboratory and the couple were isolating in their apartment. The PHL wasn't yet online, but the NYS Wadsworth Center was. The Health Police agreed to drive the samples to Albany and while we waited for the results I spoke with the couple. They returned to the States on February 24. The wife's symptoms began the evening of February 27 with congestion, muscle aches, and cough. Her husband became ill the following day with fewer, malaise, and cough. They reported that several relatives in their home country had cold symptoms, one of whom was a healthcare worker. None of the sick relatives had been tested for COVID-19. I retraced their movements in NYC for the two days before onset. They did the typical stuff—a trip for groceries, an Uber ride back to the apartment, they went up and down their building elevator and made a trip to their hospital emergency department—but had not resumed their duties.

Ordinarily, lab test results go back to the ordering physician who then notifies the patient. Governor Cuomo demanded that specimens tested at the state lab be reported to him first, of dubious ethics and legality. Cuomo convened a press conference to announce that New York State had its first COVID-19 case. This was how the wife learned that she had COVID-19. Oddly, the husband, whose symptoms were more intense, had tested negative. I figured it was likely a false negative, perhaps a poor specimen, but it didn't matter, we considered him a case, ensured that both were isolated, and planned to re-test them, but this time at PHL.

I was not privy to City Hall's reaction to the news, but I suspect it wasn't good. I then learned that Demetre and the commissioner were insisting that the hospital arrange the retesting.

The hospital's administration and head of infection control pushed back. Justifiably, they didn't want the couple to leave their apartment and risk exposing others in the building, the community, and also healthcare workers. I agreed. An impasse arose and Demetre sent staff to get me to convince the hospital to accede to the request. It dawned on me that since both were healthcare workers, they could swab each other. I offered to bring them the test kits.

I took the subway to the PHL on First Avenue where lab staff put together the test kits. Then headed uptown to the apartment. I tried to look nonchalant as I waited outside the building with a cooler in one hand and a plastic bag with the requisition forms in the other. I texted the wife to say I had arrived and to ask her to alert the doorman that they were expecting a food delivery. Yeah, it's a bit cloak and dagger, more Pink Panther-ish, but we were desperate to maintain patient confidentiality. I entered the building, but the doorman wasn't aware of any food delivery and asked me which restaurant I was from. I hadn't thought the subterfuge through and panicked. It wasn't my neighborhood, and I didn't look like the typical delivery person. I replied that I was from the diner and waved arbitrarily out the door. He looked at me and then showed me to the elevator. I left the supplies outside the couple's door, knocked three times—the agreed-upon signal—and then jogged down the hallway so we'd have no physical contact. I then waited. I heard the door open and close. Fifteen minutes later, I heard the door open and close again. I hurriedly put on gloves and retrieved the specimens, then exited the building carrying just as much as when I entered. Thankfully, the doorman didn't notice. Outside I handed the cooler to the waiting courier who transported the specimens to the PHL.

Be careful what you wish for. I had wanted to find a case,

thinking that once it was here the city would calm down. We'd been working at an insane pace. It turned out that the madness had yet to begin. Cuomo ordered the Wadsworth Center and PHL to scale up to test 1,000 specimens a day by March 9. Knowing how difficult it was for the CDC to make enough reagents; it seemed an irrational demand. The head of Health and Hospitals (H&H) complained publicly that the department refused to test their patients, neglecting to mention that we were following the CDC's criteria. The next day Demetre, during an ICS subgroup meeting, paced back and forth. He was quite animated, pointing at people like a Socratic law professor grilling students, but cutting them off before they could answer. He said that's what happens at City Hall. Others who have been on calls with the mayor confided that he often bad mouthed the department, so this came as no surprise.

I'd witnessed Demetre guzzling Red Bull, but that day he must have downed a whole case. He jumped from topic to topic—syndromic surveillance to investigating new suspect cases in the Upper West Side to anger at H&H. He vowed to go dark on H&H. Dark? He said Darth Vader-ish, dark—to cause them pain. In the next breath, he said he wasn't being vindictive but pondered filling up their isolation beds with PUIs. Marci and I looked at each other dumbfounded. That would happen soon enough without our help.

Dysfunction soon prevailed. H&H was setting up outpatient testing sites while our messaging was that if you were mildly ill, there was no need to get tested, assume it was COVID-19, stay home, and isolate. We didn't want people to risk exposing others, in a cab, on the subway, or the bus. And we especially didn't want to expose healthcare workers. If you have no symptoms, don't take resources away from those that are severely ill. Every test not only required reagents but also that healthcare workers wear personal protective equipment (PPE). Resources not already scarce would soon be.

The repeat COVID-19 test results on the couple were the same. She was positive and he was negative. It didn't fully make sense. We continued to test them long after they'd recovered and were no longer infectious and kept getting the same results. They had to return to work but couldn't as long as one of them remained positive. It was another glitch caused by political interference. The PCR test doesn't measure live virus, and positives can persist for weeks after recovery. It was foolish to keep testing them, but we were forced to keep at it. Eventually she tested negative and went back to work, and her life. They were quickly forgotten, as more cases stacked up.

Next there was a confirmed case outside NYC in neighboring Westchester County, but the man worked in the city. City Hall pressured the commissioner to release information about the patient which allowed the NYPD to go to his office building and wrap the floor in yellow crime scene tape. Not the way to prevent panic. The patient's son attended college in the city, and I was sent to the school to advise them on operational decisions. Two mayoral staffers were sitting in the back of the conference room as I spoke with the college administrators. They reported back that my advice didn't align with hizzoner's. I applied my experience, knowledge, and common sense to the unprecedented situation. Soon enough, exposures from the Westchester case spilled over into the Bronx. A school-aged child tested positive and the mayor, in his March 9 press conference, revealed enough information that the child's community identified her. The child became the target of abuse from classmates and the community. The mayor could have only obtained the information from the health commissioner or Demetre. We were outraged and vowed not to share any information that could repeat the cruelty we witnessed. The episode also seeded distrust with our departmental leadership.

The first COVID-19 wave took off in NYC in mid-March 2020, about the same time that commercial testing became available. At the peak, there were more than 6,000 cases per day. Hospitals were overburdened, as was the OCME. Rates in NYC's communities of color exceeded 1,500 cases per 100,000 population, about 60% higher than among predominantly White communities. Likewise, hospitalizations and deaths were twice as high in communities of color. Images appeared in the media of funeral homes storing bodies in cardboard coffins and refrigerator trucks parked outside hospitals. Schools closed on March 16 and the lockdown of non-essential businesses followed while hospital workers, paramedics, firefighters, police, sanitation, and MTA workers continued to go to work, as did grocery clerks and delivery persons.

D✪D Muhammad Iftekharuddin died of COVID-19 in April, as did my father, who was living in a Westchester County nursing home. Muhammad had been a D✪D longer than I had been. He was kind, soft spoken, and eternally optimistic. It was an emotionally trying time for all of us, compounded by City Hall's relentless bullying. Every cough and sniffle caused New Yorkers to bristle, shudder, and walk in the opposite direction. Then the health commissioner, under pressure from City Hall, issued an order to all City employees who were teachers, physicians, and first responders—police, fire, and EMS—that they must test negative for COVID-19 before returning to work. It was insane. There wasn't enough testing capacity in the entire United States to do this, not to mention the consumption of PPE, which was in short supply. And who would obtain the tests? Healthcare workers had more important tasks to do. What lab could handle over 100,000 tests in time to get the critical workers back on the job? Who would pay for it? Taxpayers no doubt. Yet another optical delusion.

Leaders who weren't panicking were lying. President Trump told the American public that the virus was no worse than the flu, was under control, and would miraculously go away. When it came to masks, he said they were voluntary and that he wouldn't wear one. Across the country, people harassed and attacked public health officials for doing their jobs. Harassers came to workers' homes, sent awful emails, and issued death threats. Many healthcare and public health workers quit; others retired early or were fired. Trump contracted COVID-19 during the second wave. It wasn't disclosed to the public at the time, but his oxygen levels dropped to concerning levels and he came close to needing mechanical ventilation while at Walter Reed National Military Medical Center. COVID-19 messaging was unhelpful and would get worse, as would the political interference.

The sentinel surveillance program we worked hard to set up was repeatedly delayed by City Hall. Health Alerts, the communication system created by Marci Layton to inform medical providers of the latest information about health conditions, were held up for weeks as wording kept getting changed. Perhaps the most egregious act happened shortly after the end of the first wave. The mayor announced in late May that the city would perform contact tracing of COVID-19 cases to implement isolation and quarantine. And that the responsibility of this monumental task would be that of H&H, the city agency that operates public hospitals and clinics.

We at the health department certainly didn't have all the

answers. But what we did have was decades of experience with viral respiratory diseases and a world-respected influenza expert. We had prepared a citywide plan to combat pandemic influenza and lived through H1N1, MERS, and SARS. We'd been doing contact tracing for hepatitis A, TF, and meningococcal disease for decades. A wealth of expertise additionally resided with our colleagues who had routinely performed difficult contact tracing for their target diseases—measles, syphilis, and tuberculosis. We regularly consulted with colleagues at the CDC and across the country. We read, got asked to review, and wrote research articles. To discount the D❂Ds as the mayor did was not only foolish but also the height of hubris and the apex of arrogance. Do you know who else sidelined public health and disregarded experts during the COVID-19 pandemic? Donald Trump. When challenged or faced with a knowledge deficiency, despots resort to authoritarianism.

It was as if the notoriously cantankerous former owner of the NY Yankees, George Steinbrenner, out of anger at the manager, decided to replace the entire team with professional soccer players. Skilled athletes, but not baseball players. The mayor was roundly criticized from all sides, but he stubbornly refused to relent and admit he made a mistake. Test and Trace (T2) was born, and chaos ensued, but the facade presented to the public was that everything was going smoothly. A rigid database was created to handle the work, but there weren't fields built for the needed information so producing reports was difficult and limited. Contact tracers were hired, minimally trained, and poorly supervised as the supervisors themselves had no experience in contact tracing, isolation, or quarantine. Patients were called multiple times by different contact tracers and lost patience when wrong and conflicting recommendations were issued. Workarounds were a daily requirement and the need to transfer patient data between the department and T2 caused unnecessary delays. Work that the mayor promised T2 would do better was handed back to the department when H&H failed. The mayor neglected to mention this at press conferences. One of the tasks returned to the department was the investigations of COVID-19 clusters at schools and worksites, collectively called facilities.

Although the first wave had ended and case counts were at their lowest, between 200–300 per day, we had had enough of being disrespected, ignored, and bullied. On too many conference calls I had to bite my tongue as Demetre kowtowed, capitulated, and repeatedly asked the mayoral flunkey, his chief tormentor, and public health know-nothing, "Is that right?" It was bruising to hear our expertise demeaned. It came to a head when City Hall demanded that we produce a daily report on the facilities we had investigated. We agreed to a weekly report, explaining that the investigations took time, were of historic interest, and not particularly informative to the response. Overall, people got COVID-19, went to work anyway, mistaking the symptoms for something else, and then infected coworkers. The larger issue was that our data staff was physically and emotionally exhausted. Some were on vacation, and we sought to protect them from useless busy work. On a typical day, the following reports were produced:

7:18 Daily Syndromic Surveillance Dashboard (Standard report)

8:00 Syndromic Surveillance COVID-19 alert (ED mentions of key words: travel ban countries, coronavirus)

8:02 Syndromic ILI and Pneumonia Slides (ILI+PNE counts, ILI+PNE admission counts, M-F)

8:17 FDNY EMS Syndromic Dashboard (Standard 9-1-1

call report)
8:56 Syndromic COVID-19 Daily Report (ILI+PNE counts,
*   ILI+PNE admission counts and age-stratified, M-F)*
10:02 AM COVID Case Summary Table (descriptive con-
*   firmed case table, outbreak curve by report date)*
10:17 Map of Case Count by Neighborhood
13:06 Pharmacy Prescriptions Syndromic (Tamiflu sales)
13:13 Respiratory Panel ED ILI Syndromic summary
18:02 PM Summary Table (descriptive confirmed case table,
*   outbreak curve by report date)*

City Hall dug in on the demand and Marci and I were called
to a conference call with Demetre and Commissioner Barbot. We
explained our position, half expecting that reason would prevail.
We were ordered to produce the report. We stood our ground and
refused. It wasn't just the principle but the well-being of our over-
worked staff that was at stake. We had reached the proverbial line
in the sand and were threatened to be charged with insubordina-
tion. Marci faced dismissal. My fate, since I was in civil service,
would likely be less severe. We held firm. Demetre had others
craft a workaround to satiate City Hall and less than two weeks
later, Commissioner Barbot resigned, upon request by the mayor.
Her replacement was a person from H&H with no measurable
public health experience, certainly not enough to lead an agency
as large as the department during a pandemic, but who would be
loyal and unquestioningly follow orders. To my jaundiced eye, a
puppet commissioner.

City Hall continued to hound us for data for optics, not
for decision-making. My fellow D✪Ds created a website inter-
face with real-time data that served as a model for other health
departments, but hypocritically, City Hall hemmed, hawed, and

prevaricated for weeks before approving it. Mayoral staff bullied, yelled at, and threatened departmental staff. Demetre received the brunt of the abuse, but it trickled down and affected everyone. He showed me the texts on his phone. They were relentless demands and threats that if we didn't immediately comply with every request, it would get spun up to the mayor. Our chief City Hall tormentor visited the office one day, strolling the hallways with Demetre, all smiles and insincere praise. I decided to keep one of those airplane vomit bags at my desk in the event she ever returned.

More than once Demetre was close to tears. Persons with no public health knowledge or experience were put in decision-making roles by the mayor. They led meetings, spoke ignorantly about public health, misinterpreted protocols and tenants, while they glibly uttered vacuous phrases such as, "We need to land more of these planes," "It's agnostic to how we slice it," and "We're getting good at Whac-A-Mole."

The getting good at Whac-A-Mole was a particularly misguided and blasphemous statement. Whac-A-Mole is an arcade game where plastic moles pop up through holes in a game board. The contestant attempts to whack mole heads with a mallet before they retreat into their holes. As a metaphor, Whac-A-Mole denotes an exercise in futility, not a proven public health strategy. Rather, it's a haphazard, ineffective solution to a problem for optics. The governor abused the same metaphor in a press conference as he proudly explained the second pre-wave COVID-19 approach. Cases show up in one part of the state, and you whack them. They show up in another part of the state, and you whack them. The only thing being whacked were public health workers. Cuomo might as well have said his plan was as unsinkable as the Titanic. If we asked Sisyphus to trade places with us, I expect he wouldn't. Rolling a rock perpetually up a hill is preferable to being browbeat while being forced to run in circles I suppose.

Testing was a sore spot during the pandemic. Early on there was a severe shortage of testing supplies which hampered the nation's ability to detect cases, particularly in NYC. Had we found cases two, three, or four weeks earlier than we did, would it have changed the course of the pandemic? Difficult to say. There was tremendous reluctance to shut down the city. Conceivably, had we shut down the city earlier the pandemic curve might have been flatter, but in the end, since we had no vaccine, the end result likely wouldn't have been much different. The shortage of initial testing, however, cemented in many minds that more testing was the solution. If we could ramp up testing, we'd be able to gain control of the virus. In theory, the concept has a modicum of merit. Sick or not, you get tested. The results return within twenty-four hours and if you are positive, you isolate and get called the same day as your test result so you can share the names of all your close contacts. The contacts are then called the same day and immediately placed into voluntary quarantine and monitored. Public health has used this approach for decades, with more or less success, for numerous diseases, typically one or a few cases at a time. Some examples include a single case of imported measles, hepatitis A in a food handler, and tuberculosis in a high school student. The ideal timeline rarely occurs. Neither does the full disclosure of contacts. None of these best-case-scenario contingencies were true for COVID-19.

One of the chief supporters of contact tracing was former NYC Health Commissioner Dr. Tom Frieden. Dr. Frieden also led the Bureau of Tuberculosis during the surge in cases in the 1990s. But contact tracing for tuberculosis (TB) is quite different than it is for viruses, specifically COVID-19. Very few who are exposed to TB become infectious to others and when they do it takes weeks, sometimes years, not days.

Calls for more testing got louder and louder. First just for some people, like city workers. Then for all school-aged children. Then for everyone, as often as possible. Nearly everyone with a microphone, a bullhorn, or a pulpit was echoing the sentiment. As if testing were a magic mirror that you could gaze into and know not just that you had COVID-19, but whether or not you were contagious. It was a reshaping of the Hans Christian Andersen parable, *The Emperor's New Clothes*. An illusion, or more apropos, an optical delusion.

The second wave, caused by the delta SARS-CoV-2 variant, arrived in NYC in late September/early October of 2020 and lasted through April 2021. It differed from the first wave in that it was more spread out with fewer deaths. T2, which began in June, was fully operational at the start of the second wave. Vaccines became available in December 2020 and first targeted persons at greatest risk of severe outcomes.

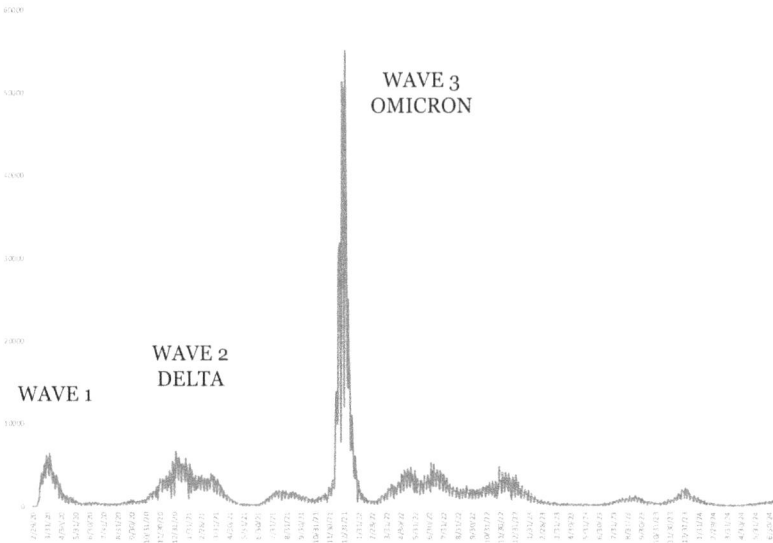

COVID-19 Cases by Day, March 2020–July 2024

Just after the new year, amid the delta wave, Marci Layton sent an email to Dr. Anthony Fauci at the National Institutes of Health. Vaccination uptake was far below expectation and her concern was the overemphasis on contact tracing was detracting from our best tool to control the pandemic. We already had the sense that contact tracing was having little, if any effect. The daily case count exceeded 6,000 on January 5, 2021, the highest single-day value to date. The media picked up on the story and questioned the spending of $880 million on the T2 program.[115]

The worst wave thus far was caused by the omicron variant. It arrived late in 2021 and lasted until February 2022. Omicron reached NYC at a time when T2 had been in operation for nineteen months, vaccine had been available for over a year, and testing availability was no longer an issue. At its height, omicron caused over 55,000 cases in a single day.[116]

Why did universal testing fail to curtail the COVID-19 pandemic? Recall that people infected with COVID-19 are believed to be contagious two days prior to symptoms, and that some people never develop symptoms. Also, that testing by itself doesn't prevent future cases from occurring. That is the role of isolation and quarantine. At the height of the first wave, a person with a cough and sore throat was presumed to have COVID-19 and told to isolate, test or no test. By recommending that everyone, ill or not, get routinely and repeatedly tested, we overloaded the still-developing laboratory capacity. As a result, reagent supplies dwindled, and turnaround times (TAT) increased to as long as a week. The data produced by T2 showed that the mean number of days from SAR-CoV-2 sample collection to receipt to assign for interview in August 2020 hit a peak of nine days. Now, add to that the two days the person was infectious before symptom onset and you can clearly see the system was too slow to stop, or slow, COVID-19 transmission even while case counts were at their lowest.

At the beginning of the delta wave, the TAT decreased to six days, but it was still not fast enough to affect the pandemic curve. Overall, the focus on testing had huge detrimental implications. It resulted in congregate care facilities being in the same queue as people who wanted testing so they could safely take a trip. All the testing used up precious reagents and PPE and placed health-care workers, as well as the general population, at unnecessary risk by sending infected people out of their homes to get tested. To protect others the message should have been, if you are sick, stay home. Knowing for certain that your symptoms were due to COVID-19 was a luxury that only fueled the pandemic. The mean TAT eventually reached four days, still longer than model-ers predicted would be effective. But the testing delay wasn't the only problem faced by the T2 program.

Another problem with the test-everyone-often policy was that the gold-standard test, PCR, is quite sensitive, but does not identify persons who are infectious. PCR cannot discriminate between live/infectious and dead/non-infectious virus. In fact, we learned early on during the pandemic that PCR tests can remain positive for weeks even months after the illness has resolved. So, a person who perhaps had mild or no symptoms early during the pandemic when tests weren't available, who then decided to get tested as recommended and was positive, posed no risk to anyone. However, they were subjected to isolation and their family members to quarantine. And who bore the burden of all the testing? People in low-income communities who neither had paid sick leave nor the flexibility to work from home. Data from the first wave in NYC revealed that rates of COVID-19 were two times higher in the very high versus lowest poverty categories.

There had been a core of seasoned departmental epidemiologists who repeatedly said that we can't test our way out of the pandemic. The tests, when they became available, weren't perfect. The antigen test required a greater level of virus to be present than PCR. This meant that even if everyone was able to get tested daily, as impractical as it was, it wouldn't be enough. That's because a person who tested negative by antigen before they left their home for work or school in the morning might be contagious in the afternoon when they got on the subway to go home. The tests created a false sense of security.

And what of the false positive tests? The tests are for the purpose of making a diagnosis. This means the person being tested has symptoms compatible with the illness and a high likelihood of disease, known as the pre-test probability. Testing people without any symptoms, otherwise known as screening, wasn't how the tests were designed. Screening doesn't work the same as diagnosis. It will give many more false positives, and those people will be required to remain at home when they needn't. It has to do with the pre-test probability, or the amount of disease anticipated in the population to be tested.

There's an exercise that's taught in entry-level epidemiology that demonstrates the role of pre-test probability. Suppose that the COVID-19 test has a sensitivity of 95%, meaning that if you test 100 people with COVID-19 the test will be positive in ninety-five people, which is very good. On the flip side, the test is 90% specific, which means if you test 100 people who don't have COVID-19 the test will be negative in ninety of them, also a respectable number. The exercise then applies this test to two hypothetical populations. The first is a group of 100 people who have a reason to believe they might have COVID-19; either they have compatible symptoms, live with, or have had close contact with a known case. Let's set the true value of COVID-19 in this population at 40%. Some of these people will have other illnesses, perhaps another respiratory virus like influenza or a non-infectious cause of their symptoms. The test will correctly identify thirty-eight of the forty as having COVID-19 and will miss just two. Testing this population will wrongly identify six people as having COVID-19 who don't. I think we can live with that.

For the second population, instead of people who have a reason to suspect COVID-19, we decided to test the general population, and for this exercise, it will be one million people. In this group, the probability of having COVID-19 is much lower, say 5%. If we apply the same test, we will correctly diagnose 47,500 persons with COVID-19 out of the actual 50,000 infected, but we will also misdiagnose 95,000 people as having COVID-19 when they don't. That's a huge number of false positives and the consequences are not innocuous. These positives are sent for contact tracing, overburdening the system, not to mention the trouble brought to families by having to isolate and quarantine.

The abilities of PCR and rapid antigen tests to correctly diagnose SARS-CoV-2 when present and when not present differ. PCR does better when patients are symptomatic, but less well when they aren't—meaning high sensitivity but lower specificity. Rapid antigen is the opposite—lower sensitivity but higher specificity. This complicates testing, but regardless, if contact tracing can't act quickly enough or keep up when case counts rise, then massive testing is a waste of money and more importantly, of testing resources. Early in the second wave, laboratories got overwhelmed and their TAT increased. This illustrates the mistake of using a diagnostic test on the wrong population. But this is exactly what the mayor did.

Who benefited from all the testing? Laboratories did.

Labcorp's net profits increased from $824 million in 2019 to $1.56 billion in 2020 and $2.4 billion in 2021.[117] Quest Diagnostics's profits increased from $858 million in 2019 to $1.43 billion in 2020 and $1.99 billion in 2021.[118] Their stock prices also rose. Labcorp by 78% and Quest by 56% when comparing closing prices on 1/3/2020 to 1/3/2022.[119,120] I wonder how many of the armchair epidemiologists who jumped on the testing bandwagon were invested in these companies or were on their payrolls?

The early symptoms of COVID-19, a runny nose, muscle aches, and sore throat, are neither specific to coronavirus nor uncommon. When these symptoms first began, many people considered alternative diagnoses such as allergies, insufficient sleep, or overdoing it at the gym. Getting tested during the early pandemic waves required leaving home which we advised people with COVID-19 against. Once a test was obtained, it took time to transport the sample to the laboratory, perform the test, confirm the result, enter the result into the laboratory computer system, and report to the health department. The health department then had to process the data, remove the duplicates, and transfer the data to T2. Once the report was received by T2, the case was placed in the queue awaiting an investigator/contact tracer. Depending on the volume of cases, it might sit in the queue for hours or even days. If the file contained a correct phone number several attempts were made to reach the person. If there wasn't a number or it was incorrect, efforts were made to obtain a correct number. This timeline hampered T2's effectiveness and only worsened as the volume of cases grew.

In my observation and analysis, contact tracing in NYC was ineffective at slowing transmission of COVID-19. Anyone who claims differently is putting lipstick on a pig. It's still a pig and won't pass as your date to the Met Gala. The evidence comes from two sources: T2's own data and by comparing the second and third pandemic waves to the first.

Trace's data for the period of June 1, 2020–December 31, 2021, reveals that they received 1,252,586 COVID-19 cases to process and that two-thirds completed intake and 38% completed monitoring. During the omicron wave, the percentage who completed intake dropped to 41%, just over half provided contacts, and for the entire period, there were 1.1 contacts elicited per case, and 27% completed monitoring. By comparison, Taiwan reported identifying 17 contacts per case, the United Kingdom 2, and France 1.4.

I compared the first wave when no contact tracing was in place, to the second wave when contact tracing was in place. I defined the first wave as February 29–June 30, 2020, and it occurred when no one had immunity to the virus. There were 218,570 cases and 22,959 deaths. A total of 1,765,889 COVID-19 tests were performed, mostly on symptomatic persons, and there was no contact tracing, monitoring, or systematic communication with contacts about quarantining. Mask-wearing and social distancing improved over the four months but by no means were they universal.

I defined the start and end dates of the second wave as October 1, 2020, and March 31, 2021, respectively. The second wave lasted longer and infected 610,927 persons, more than twice as many as the first wave. Far fewer persons died, 7,808, in part because the curve was flatter, which relieved the stress on the healthcare system. We also had better treatments. But why was the curve flatter? Approximately 24% of the population had some immunity from the first wave, masks reduced exposure as well as the amount of virus a person inhaled which lessened disease severity. Social distancing had similar effects. The number of COVID-19 tests performed during the second wave was 10,618,908 and the testing of people without any symptoms was common. We also learned that some people avoided getting tested during the second wave so that their names would not be reported by labs. Whether they isolated and their contacts quarantined or not is speculative. So, what effect can we directly attribute to contact tracing? Since testing was limited in the first wave, it is likely the actual case count was higher, but despite this, I fail to see much of an effect that can be attributed to the estimated billion dollars spent on testing and contact tracing. This doesn't account for the dispro-portionate effect on low-income communities where working from home was not an option and neither was not working.

Now let's turn to omicron, the third wave. One look at the COVID-19 cases-by-day graph should be enough to cast seri-ous doubt on the effectiveness of T2 to slow, stall, impede, or put a dent in the pandemic's path. Some may argue it wasn't a fair fight. That the rate of new cases in the second wave simply overwhelmed T2. Here's the rub with that argument. T2 began operations in June 2020. Throughout the summer of 2020, there were between 200–300 cases per day. If contact tracing was truly effective wouldn't those numbers have declined? Should've there been better results with a four-month head start before the second wave? What about the nineteen months of advanced preparation before the third wave? Wasn't that enough time to show value for the money spent? The best we can say about T2 is that if case counts are low, it, along with social distancing, masking, and sev-eral lockdown measures, can temporarily maintain case counts at that level. However, it was about as useful during the second and third pandemic waves as using teaspoons to bail water from the sinking Titanic. Make those diamond-encrusted, gold teaspoons.

What role did the mayor's decision to transfer the responsibil-ity of contact tracing to H&H play? By law, COVID-19 reports had to come to the health department. By shifting the responsibility of contact tracing to H&H, which had minimal experience in this regard, people with no experience had to learn a new skill. Imagine being placed in the air traffic controller tower at an airport and told to land planes. What's more, a new database had to be built from scratch. It's no surprise then that the database that was created was rigid, and developers were reluctant to make critical modifications. It also had severe limitations, one being that COVID-19 reports from the health department had to be transferred daily, adding another day to the contact tracing delay. Not that I think the department could've kept up with the volume of cases.

The T2 case prioritization was also an issue. Symptomatic persons are more worrisome as coughing and sneezing disperse more infectious particles. However, there was no way to know this from the laboratory reports or by scanning the T2 queue—another reason why testing people without symptoms clogged the system. Add to this the problem of getting accurate phone numbers; people refusing to answer calls, not completing the lengthy questionnaire, reluctance to disclose contacts, and not completing monitoring; it comes as no surprise that the system failed, despite being lauded by the mayor and his cronies.

There's a maxim in medicine. Don't order a test if you don't intend to make a decision based on the results. The correlation in epidemiology is that there isn't much value in performing an analysis if you don't have a plan to act on the results. This is especially true during emergencies where there are already a tremendous number of demands and stress on staff. But City Hall didn't have such training, knowledge, or sense. Nor did they listen. Their data requests were as relentless as they were useless. As a result, we spent numerous hours discussing metrics. And between the waves, the mayor demanded the equivalent of a smoke detector, an alarm to tell him when to get out of the building, meaning when to go back into pause/lockdown. Pandemics don't work that way. There's no on/off switch. At their request, we fiddled with different data indicators and suggested a set, only to be rejected without explanation. Weeks passed, and then we were asked the same question again, and again.

That wasn't the extent of the nonsense. The City Hall brain trust decided we should present our case rates and other numbers with two decimal places. So, the COVID-19 rate as 200.13 per 100,000, instead of 200.1 or just 200. It was plain ludicrous to suggest the extra decimal place had a level of precision, or value to people, or was of any significance whatsoever to decision-making. Imagine if you can, being a soldier fighting a battle and having to take orders from a person whose only experience with war was playing with toy soldiers.

Maybe you're thinking that all of these mistakes are clear in hindsight and faulting the decisions is Monday-morning quarterbacking. Well, long after it was shown that testing school-aged children gained very little toward slowing the pandemic, the testing continued and at great inconvenience to families and at great expense, especially for private schools since it wasn't paid for by the City. The detrimental effects of repeated exclusions and school closures on student achievement are coming to light but have yet to be fully realized. Dr. Jay Varma, a former deputy commissioner for the health department, was the primary COVID-19 adviser to the mayor. He was the chief proponent of testing, especially in schools. He was the first author on a paper published about the NYC public school testing program during the period October 9 to December 18, 2020. According to his paper, nearly a quarter of a million tests were performed on students, teachers, and staff in a randomly assigned rotation. The overall percent positivity for asymptomatic students and staff was 0.4%.[121] The paper did not include the cost of the program but concluded that the "overall burden of COVID-19 infections was no higher than the burden in the general community and that transmission within schools was not common." Despite this reassurance, testing in schools didn't end until the fall of 2022 at an estimated cost of $30 million a month.

So, what should have been the response? One could argue that all that the City did during the first three waves of COVID-19 was worth trying. But the tenacity with which the City stuck with ineffective strategies can't be justified. The greatest number of COVID-19 transmissions occurred in homes, so supporting families and small businesses would have been a good place to spend the bulk of the funds NYC received from the federal government. However, during the height of the waves, even this activity would have been overwhelming. Before the second wave hit, I pleaded with the department leadership to change our direction. To concede that we were not going to stamp out COVID-19, but perhaps we could reach a tolerable level of disease with reduced severity. I argued that contact tracing wasn't working, not for a lack of effort, funding, or testing, but because of the insurmountable barriers already listed.

As proof of my assertions, I asked if anyone knew the proportion of new COVID-19 cases who were in quarantine at the time of diagnosis. Meaning, that T2 had identified them as a contact before they became infectious, placed them in quarantine, and therefore interrupted further transmission. Jennifer Baumgartner, one of our most experienced analysts, did the calculations. For the twelve weeks from July 9 to September 19, 2020, T2 processed an average of 1,941 cases per week and the percentage placed in quarantine prior to symptom onset ranged between 1.9 and 6.5%. This revealed that over 90% of people diagnosed with COVID-19 were not already at home when they learned of their diagnosis.

The cracks in the system were larger than the floorboards. Cases slipped through like grains of sand filling the pit faster than we could dig it. My brain kept telling me that we were chasing our tails and that no amount of testing (flawed), money (wasted), or effort (misplaced) was going to change this. But City Hall was making a big show of it with lots of hand-waving and stern admonishments in press conferences. When case counts crept up for weeks before the second wave, City Hall responded by doubling down on ineffective actions. That's something out of the Trump playbook. The mayor behaved like a gambler losing at craps and thinking that his luck was going to change, failing to realize that math prevails over hope.

We wanted the health department and City Hall to pivot. People diagnosed with COVID-19 still needed to be isolated, but we needed to limit quarantine requests for household contacts only. And do a better job educating and supporting people to lessen the burden of isolation. In addition, mask use needed to be a larger part of the messaging. Perhaps I was overly optimistic, but I believed we could increase compliance if we explained how masks worked. In addition to limiting transmission, masks can decrease the inoculum or the amount of virus that enters your body, so if you do get sick, the illness would be milder. Emphasize the value of mask adherence in indoor spaces with poor ventilation and leverage community providers and organizations to spread that message. We needed to move toward a more tolerable balance of individual freedom and community protection. With all the money being thrown at testing, why not enlist celebrities and influencers to wear fashionable masks? Combatting vaccine misinformation was a more difficult communication message, but equally deserving of funding, as opposed to continuing to pour money on ineffective contact tracing.

The first report about COVID-19 in a long-term health facility involved a skilled nursing facility outside of Seattle, Washington. In the three weeks from February 22–March 9, eighty-one patients contracted COVID-19, along with thirty-four staff and fourteen visitors; twenty-one patients and one visitor died.[122] The mortality rate of 27% in patients should have been enough to guide governmental officials on how to allocate resources. At the same time, a report appeared in *The New England Journal of Medicine* detailing 171 children under sixteen years of age who were diagnosed with COVID-19 in Wuhan, China. While 65% of the children had evidence of pneumonia, only three required ICU care, all of whom had medical comorbidities. One death occurred in a ten-month-old child with a pre-existing illness for a mortality rate of 0.6%.[123] At the onset we argued for a mitigation strategy, as opposed to attempting control, to protect the most vulnerable populations such as the elderly and persons residing in congregate settings, including nursing and group homes, persons with co-morbidities who lived at home but relied on others for assistance, and support for frontline healthcare workers with adequate PPE, testing, guidance, and staffing.

Returning to the sentinel surveillance, influenza-negative specimens we had collected in early March 2020, we eventually got them tested. It came as no surprise that we found positives. We next reviewed reports from January and February 2020, when testing was restricted.

The ride-share driver, who tested positive several months after his illness by PCR and antibodies, was determined to be the earliest case with onset on January 28; a month before the first recognized case. Three other patients had onset in the first two weeks of February and thirty-five had onset in the last two weeks of the month, all before the first cases were recognized in NYC. This retrospective survey was undoubtedly an undercount of the true number of COVID-19 infections in NYC prior to February 29. There were 237 persons reported to the health department with compatible symptoms during the period who were never tested. In a study conducted by Mount Sinai Health Systems, SARS-CoV-2 RNA was identified in a patient respiratory specimen collected on January 25, before the ride-share driver.[124] COVID-19 was clearly circuiting in NYC a month before the first recognized, positive case. The delay in testing capacity resulted in delayed recognition of circulating virus, which impaired the public health response until well after community transmission was established. But the future isn't all bleak. Wastewater testing is a promising sentinel detection system that many jurisdictions are adopting and has the potential to detect a host of pathogens before they circulate widely.

Demetre Daskalakis left the department in December 2020. Marci Layton left one year later. COVID-19 never left. At the time of this writing, NYC is experiencing another COVID-19 surge and averaging about 1,000 cases per day, however, the expansion of home testing makes case counts unreliable as home tests are rarely reported.[125] In March 2022, the CDC officially recommended that health departments scale back contact tracing and focus on high-risk settings such as nursing homes and other congregate facilities. Many health departments had already abandoned contact tracing when they were overwhelmed by the omicron wave. The CDC's rationale was that there were other tools, but in reality, the practice had been expensive and exhausting, with dubious effectiveness.

The ride-share driver died in May 2021 of complications from his COVID-19 illness. His death wasn't initially classified as due to COVID-19. Marie and I worked with the family and physician to amend the death certificate. The family deserved the government's COVID-19 death benefit. Public health could have done more for all the victims of COVID-19.

CHAPTER 15

Not All Mystery Illnesses Are Infectious

Kids find trouble. When he was four years old, my youngest brother removed the side rails to his junior bed, pretended they were crutches, and promptly tumbled down the stairs. He broke his forearm. A week or so later we went out to eat and, embarrassed by the cast, he refused to go inside the restaurant. So, we sat in the car, under the El on Jerome Avenue in the Bronx, for what seemed like hours while my mother coaxed him into Peter Pan's. This led to the family saying, "I'm starving to death outside a Chinese restaurant." Years later, I treated a child in the Jacobi ED who had sucked the air out of a wide-mouthed Malta bottle creating a vacuum that trapped her tongue. Her breathing was becoming labored so we wedged a lubricated infant feeding catheter between her tongue and the bottle rim to release the vacuum. Another child swallowed a Superball, a 1970's toy rubber ball that bounces erratically, which lodged between his uvula and vocal cords. The Superball created a ball valve and required immediate removal as it impaired the child's ability to breathe. Another child who attended a carnival was struck in the back of the head by an errantly thrown dart. He was in no pain despite the dart having penetrated both the outer and inner tables of the skull. His uncle attempted removal, as evidenced by his footprint on the boy's scalp, but the dart was as embedded as Excalibur in stone. The child underwent neurosurgery. Fortunately, all the children survived. Yet trouble isn't always self-inflicted and the outcome unscathed.

So, when I was asked to assist OCME with an investigation of a three-year-old's death these incidents floated in the back of my mind. It was late May 2021, the second wave of COVID-19 was waning and NYC was looking forward to a normal summer. Deputy Chief Medical Examiner Dr. Melissa Pasquale asked if I could review the case and advise if we thought it was suspicious for an infectious death. Dr. Pasquale had been instrumental during the meningococcal outbreaks and leptospirosis cluster.

The case was tragic. A three-year-old boy died two days after being hospitalized. The presumptive diagnosis made by the hospital was the Miller Fisher variant of Guillain-Barré syndrome—the eponymous variant of an eponymous syndrome. Miller Fisher is a neurologic disorder characterized by a descending paralysis that starts with the major nerves in the head that control eye movement and then progresses downward. Like Guillain-Barré syndrome, it is a result of antibodies, formed as a result of a viral or bacterial infection, that attack your nerve cells. What Dr. Pasquale knew was that Miller Fisher syndrome mimics botulism, which is one of the reportable diseases we urgently investigate. As a result, she asked us if this was a case of concern and did we have any special work-up to recommend? Miller Fisher syndrome is rare, and I couldn't recall ever hearing about it in kids, so it immediately struck me as an odd diagnosis. Typically, patients with Miller Fisher syndrome recover in a matter of months. There was limited clinical information in Dr.Pasquale's email, so I enlisted Paula's help, and we got busy.

The boy, who I'll call Peter, had vomited three times over the course of one week. That same week, his mother took him to a doctor who prescribed an antibiotic for an inflamed throat while awaiting culture results. The day he was admitted to the hospital was different. He was less active and didn't want to eat. He arrived at the ED at about half past eight on a Monday morning. The doctors couldn't find any obvious explanation for his symptoms, so they ordered tests. It was while Peter was in radiology that additional symptoms developed that prompted the diagnosis of Miller Fisher Syndrome. Namely, he was unsteady on his feet. Unsteadiness can be caused by many ailments, but the child also had abnormalities that pointed to dysfunction of his cranial nerves. There are ten cranial nerves that control important functions such as sight, eye movements, hearing, and swallowing. Peter's eyelids were droopy, and his face didn't have the usual contours, a sign that the nerves that control those muscles were damaged. These are symptoms of botulism, hence Dr.Pasquale's concern. A neurologist was consulted who found ptosis or droopy eyelid worse in the right eye than the left, diminished facial movement, normal deep tendon reflexes, and down-going toes on plantar reflex. The sole of the foot is stroked with a firm object from heel to toe. A normal plantar reflex response is for the toes to curl down if the patient doesn't just pull away. If the toes got up instead, it suggests that the problem is in the brain.

Putting all of the physical findings together allows doctors to produce a list of differential diagnoses. On the list for this child, along with Miller Fisher variant, was encephalitis, myasthenia gravis, a brain tumor, and botulism. Tests would help determine what was causing Peter's diagnosis, but there was a fly in the ointment. A claim of medical neglect had been lodged anonymously and the Administration for Child Services (ACS) was called to investigate. It was unclear if the parents were married but they were in the middle of a custody battle. Peter was an only child and lived with his mother in a Brooklyn apartment. Peter's mother was Chinese and had stopped working in January 2021. His grandmother had moved in to help care for him. The father is African American and works in an office. He reportedly didn't have access to drugs or chemicals. Coincidentally, Peter's grandmother had died suddenly from a non-COVID-19 illness earlier in the year.

Imaging studies of Peter's brain were normal, which ruled out a tumor. The lumbar puncture and examination of spinal fluid made encephalitis or Miller Fisher unlikely as the typical findings were absent. All the tests to find a viral illness were negative, as were a battery of tests to look for the usual drug overdoses, such as aspirin, acetaminophen, and barbiturates. Cocaine, amphetamine, marijuana, and other recreational drugs were also negative. The tests for a metabolic imbalance, including liver function, were normal as was the complete blood count, which tests for anemia and evidence of a systemic infection. There was, however, one minor abnormality. The platelet count was low. The normal range for platelets is 150,000–400,000 per microliter of blood. Peter's was 160,000, which was barely above the lower limit of normal. Alone there wasn't much to make of this finding. To test for the Miller Fisher variant a special antibody test called GQ1B needed to be sent to a specialty laboratory. For myasthenia gravis, a Tensilon test, however, myasthenia gravis in a previously well three-year-old is rarer than rare. All that remained on the differential diagnoses list was botulism.

Botulism is a neurologic illness caused by a potent toxin from the bacteria *Clostridium botulinum.* The bacteria are a normal inhabitant of soil and rarely cause human illness. The botulism cases we typically see in NYC are of the infant variety, where the child, usually less than one year of age, accidentally ingests the organism and it reproduces in the intestinal tract and elaborates toxin. The children appear weak, with difficult head control, weak cries, and poor feeding. Affected infants have abnormalities of their cranial nerves and if untreated, can progress to paralysis of lung muscles and death. Three to five cases of infant botulism occur each year in NYC, but no deaths. Treatment is with an anti-toxin that is produced by one lab in the United States.

Older children and adults can prevent *C. botulinum* from growing and producing toxin in the gastrointestinal tract. The way children and adults contract botulism is by ingesting the toxin in food. Many of us learned as kids not to eat from dented cans, the reason being that *C. botulinum* produces gas that expands the tops or bottoms of tin cans. This doesn't happen much anymore, as most foodborne botulism occurs from improper home canning or preparation of fermented foods. Foodborne botulism is even rarer than infant botulism, with about one case every five years. There are two other ways botulism can occur though—through a wound contaminated with soil and by dermatologic treatments with the toxin. These are the rarest of all forms of botulism. The Wadsworth Center laboratory can diagnose botulism from a small sample of blood. The PHL uses the mouse assay, where mice are injected with a sample and then observed for botulism symptoms. If a mouse dies, they are re-injected but this time some mice get anti-toxin. If anti-toxin prevents death, then the presence of botulism toxin is confirmed.

The day after admission, just before midnight, with both mother and father at his bedside, Peter again vomited. What transpired next was likely a frenzy of activity. A nurse was summoned, and she found Peter in respiratory distress with foam coming from his mouth. She called a code and ushered the parents to a waiting area. For more than two hours the code team worked to resuscitate him. They placed an endotracheal tube to provide oxygen directly to Peter's lungs. Fluid was then administered to bolster his blood pressure and cardiac drugs were administered to speed up his heart rate which had dropped dangerously low. Unlike adults, the heart in children is quite resilient. It speeds up when the blood pressure is low, and only slows down when there isn't enough oxygen to keep it beating. Peter had bradycardia, a slower than normal heart rate, and he wasn't responding to the usual medications. The code team ordered a portable x-ray machine which took a chest image at the bedside, but no answer was found. The lungs looked clear, and the heart appeared to be normal size. Inexplicably, Peter's heart rate remained low and just after 2 a.m., he died.

The autopsy did not reveal the cause of death. Specimens were obtained for routine tests and saved for as-yet-to-be-determined tests. While Dr. Pasquale interviewed the parents, Paula and I combed through the medical and OCME records. There was one finding during the autopsy that gave Paula and me pause. On the right anterior thigh was a wound that according to the child's mother had not been present before hospitalization.

We examined the digital photo. The wound was circular, a little larger than a half an inch in diameter, and was surrounded by a reddish-purple ring, as you might see in a fresh bruise. The skin overlying the center of the wound was intact and dark gray, with a thin, whitish circumferential ring. A small, raised area near the margin resembled a blister, though it was hard to be certain from the single photographic image. There was no dried blood or scab.

A plausible explanation was found in the chart—an order had been written to administer a flu vaccine to the child. But when I inquired about this with one of the intensive care doctors, I was told no vaccine had been given, furthermore, no documentation of the wound existed in the hospital chart. In addition, there was no mention of the wound in the physician's physical exam notes nor in the nursing notes.

I stared at the photo. It was taken postmortem so I considered what influence that might have had on what I was seeing. The dark gray was almost black, and it suggested an eschar, from the Greek, *eskhara*, which means charcoal hearth. Two diseases that feature eschars immediately came to mind, Rickettsialpox, a mouse mite-transmitted disease, and anthrax. The latter can be fatal, but the child's clinical course did not fit with either. I have never seen a case of wound botulism, but a related bacterium, *Clostridium perfringens*, causes gangrene, a black-colored necrosis of the skin. Botulism can progress to respiratory muscle paralysis which might explain what happened to the child. Paula did the hard part, locating specimens, completing the necessary paperwork, and arranging shipment of serum, stool, and wound tissue to the Wadsworth Center in Albany to test for botulism.

I didn't think it was botulism. Peter never had lower extremity muscle weakness which should occur before trouble breathing, although he did have ataxia. It also seemed that he progressed from respiratory to cardiac arrest too fast. No postmortem findings in his lungs suggested that he had aspirated, which could have occurred when he vomited. We got negative results from the tissue and stool for the botulinum toxins A, B, F, and F by MALDI-TOF the following week. And although the blood vial leaked and could not be tested, the other results were negative for botulism. The Wadsworth Center kept trying to use enrichment broth to coax *C. botulinum* to grow, but with no luck.

Dr. Pasquale interviewed Peter's parents about the events leading up to his illness. The custody battle was over parenting styles. The mother felt the father was too cavalier, allowing the child to play dangerously. While the father accused the mother of not attending to medical care expediently. ACS was now involved in the custody dispute and the father was only allowed visits at a third-party location. The last time Peter spent time with him was on May 18. On that day, Peter was his usual active self, playing, running, and jumping. He didn't eat anything but drank water from a bottle his mother sent with him. Peter vomited on the way home, but this was after he left his father's company. The father told Dr. Pasquale that he wanted her to take him for medical evaluation. The next day, though he admitted his recall may be faulty, the father had a video call with his son and noted him to be stumbling around, which he thought was unusual. He again asked that she take him to be seen by a doctor. When asked about the thigh injury, Peter's father noted it the day after hospital admission when Peter returned from getting an MRI.

The day before Peter was admitted to the hospital, he ate store-bought shrimp dumplings, spareribs, and homemade congee. He was prescribed amoxicillin for a sore throat and began the medication on the same day. On the day of admission, Peter didn't want to eat or drink. While waiting in the ED, Peter's mother tried to give him cookies, but he spit them out. Peter was in the hospital for less than three days and his mother stated she was with him the entire time, except when she met with a social worker. During that meeting, Peter's father was with him.

I received an email from Dr. Gaffoor, the director of pediatric ICU at the hospital. It had an attachment. It is typical in fatal cases for hospitals to review the case. He got my contact information from the ICU doctor I had spoken with and was contacting me to share their thoughts on what had transpired. During the code an x-ray had been taken, the first and only one during the admission. The x-ray did not show any lung or heart pathology but curiously revealed what looked like retained contrast in the stomach. Contrast is used to enhance the visualization of tissues during several radiography procedures; however, the hospital had no record of giving contrast and asked if the contents could be analyzed.

The image attached to the email appeared as a thumbnail, and I clicked on it to view the full image. Solid things, like bones, block the x-rays from reaching the film and appear white while the air-filled lungs appear black. Just below the left lung, in the anatomical location of the stomach, there was a half-moon shaped object, occupying about one-quarter the width of his torso. The image color was a brighter white and scalloped in appearance, reminiscent of swirling cream in a cup of coffee. A trail of material exited from the bottom left and disappeared below the edge of the radiograph. Dr. Gaffoor also shared that the neurology team thought that the sudden cardiac collapse raised the prospect of a metabolic or mitochondrial/genetic disorder. I shared the radiograph finding with Dr. Pasquale, who was already aware as she saw a faint coating of material when she had examined the child's stomach but didn't know what to make of it. The material was scant, and none had been saved for testing.

There were several inconsistencies in the medical record. In addition to the order to give the child an influenza vaccine, which I was assured by the intensive care doctors was not given, the thigh wound wasn't mentioned in the notes, despite the doctor telling me she had seen it and questioned the mother about it. The date the child began the terminal event was written in the chart as

May 26, when it was actually May 25. It wasn't a stretch to imagine that the child could have received contrast, either intentionally
or by accident. I considered what else might give this appearance
seen on the radiograph and could cause the constellation of symptoms Peter had. Heavy metals came to mind.

My first job in public health was in childhood lead poisoning prevention. Acute lead toxicity can cause gastrointestinal
distress as well as neurologic symptoms. Peeling lead paint chips
are sweet and often the source of childhood poisoning, but NYC
had removed most lead from apartments. But in an old building,
there could be sources of lead. Another heavy metal that would
appear radiopaque is bismuth, an ingredient in Pepto Bismol, an
over-the-counter medication used for gastrointestinal illnesses.
Could this have been given to the child by a parent? Other heavy
metals that came to mind were mercury, polonium, and thallium,
the latter two had been used by the Soviet Union to attack foes.
Chloral hydrate, a medicine used for sedation, is also radiopaque.
The child had brain imaging so perhaps sedation was given to get
a good image. Both the hospital and parents denied giving Pepto
Bismol and no order for chloral hydrate was written in the chart.
Further complicating the issue is that the contrast was only seen
in the stomach, and a trace in the duodenum, the part of the small
intestine that the stomach empties into. Dr. Pasquale explained
that when mixed with stool further down the tract it becomes less
concentrated and harder to distinguish on radiograph.

When the medical examiner takes jurisdiction over an
investigation it is their staff, the physician pathologist, who com-
municates with the family and unless requested to do so, BCD
rarely intercedes. Medical examiner investigations are methodical, detailed, and thorough. What they aren't is fast. Most BCD
investigations have a shorter timeline. We're looking for ongoing

exposures to stop so others don't get sick. That urgency to prevent ongoing exposures sometimes comes up with joint BCD-OCME investigations, but it can't speed up their processes. After a thorough examination of the body and organs, tissue samples are sent for histological examination. Specimens from all major organs, including the brain, are fixed in a preservative, stained, and carefully examined under a microscope. Histology provides clues, but rarely a specific diagnosis. Yet it can guide further diagnostic testing. However, this process takes weeks to complete. In the meantime, Dr. Pasquale summarized in a series of emails what she learned from conversations with the child's parents. Bottom line: nothing stood out. But I knew I likely didn't have all the facts. It seemed like a toxin. Perhaps a folk remedy? Containing digitalis? Digitalis would cause bradycardia.

Curiously, in her repeated conversations with Peter's mother, she asked Dr. Pasquale if it could be lead poisoning. Acute lead poisoning was quite prevalent in cities due to the use of lead in paint and leaded gasoline. Significant progress has been made over the last fifty years to reduce the prevalence of lead poisoning, but it still occurs. The mother's persistence struck Dr. Pasquale as odd. The heavy metal test panel wasn't routine, but as she was out of avenues to pursue, she packaged specimens and sent them to be tested. The OCME heavy metal test panel included arsenic, antimony, barium, bismuth, lead, mercury, selenium, and thallium. Dr. Pasquale had been given a water bottle by the mother, allegedly the one from Peter's last visit with his father. She logged it in and placed it in the freezer, just in case.

Several weeks later the histology report was completed, and I was most interested in the thigh wound findings. There was evidence of acute inflammation, and the breakdown of fat cells—all in all, nonspecific signs. There wasn't any gross or microscopic bleeding to suggest there had been an injection, however, the pathologist was careful to not rule one out. The thigh wound remained unexplained and by all accounts, it did not appear until day two of hospitalization. The remainder of the histology report was unremarkable. Nothing was found in the heart to explain Peter's sudden cardiac collapse. Still pending was the neuropathology report.

One more detail would surface before the case went temporarily cold. A radiograph taken by the OCME of Peter's thigh, at the site of the wound, also showed radiopaque material. This meant someone had injected him. The investigation changed entirely. Up to now, Peter's death could have been the result of an accidental ingestion. Now it was leaning towards a homicide investigation.

With this new information, Peter's grandmother's death was revisited. She had taken ill in February 2021 and vomited after preparing her lunch. She described whole-body numbness and presented to the emergency room the following day. Doctors thought she might have been having a stroke, but tests proved negative. Per Peter's mother, her cardiac enzymes were very high and was presumed to have had a cardiac event. She died that afternoon. No autopsy was performed, and the exact cause of death was not determined.

In August, the neuropathologist submitted Peter's report to Dr. Pasquale. Her findings were most consistent with an autoimmune illness affecting the nervous system. Autoimmune means that your body is triggered to make antibodies to attack your own tissues. Multiple sclerosis is an example of an autoimmune neurologic illness. The test for antibodies found in Miller Fisher variant, however, had been negative. The neuropathologist wrote that she didn't think the findings were the result of a toxin. Another month passed and in mid-September, Dr. Pasquale called. She was typically professional and reserved, but on this call, she was not her usual self. Excited, anxious, disturbed, it was hard to tell which. The news was about Peter and was too sensitive to put in an email. The lab had found high levels of thallium!

The element thallium has an atomic number of eighty-one and sits in the Periodic Table row between mercury and lead, three removed from polonium—a veritable murder's row of the elements. In its pure form, it is a gray to silvery metal, and thallium compounds have found use as rat poisons and insecticides. Thallium was banned for commercial use in the United States in 1975 but still has industrial uses in the semiconductor industry. Thallium remains legal in other countries. Thallium compounds are odorless and tasteless and have been the chemical of choice of poisoners. It requires no expertise to use other than figuring out the lethal dose. Due to structural similarities, the human body handles thallium as if it were potassium. Wherever physiologic processes rely on potassium, thallium's poisonous effects are found. It will disrupt the heart rhythm, destroy the nerve protein myelin, and interfere with energy production. Thallium levels less than two micrograms per liter (μ/L) are considered normal. This is because anything in our environment can find its way into our bodies. This level is too low to cause toxic effects, that level is greater than 200 μ/L in blood. The amount of thallium found in Peter's blood was more than 500 μ/L.

In 1935 Coney Island, low-wage bookkeeper Frederick Gross, the sole supporter of a family of eight, was accused of murder. Four of his five children and his wife were determined to have been poisoned by thallium-contaminated cocoa. His mother-in-law and one son survived. Gross was known to his neighbors as a kind and gentle soul. No one could believe he could have committed such a crime. As Gross sat in jail, investigators probed his life, finding no motive or purchase of the poison. When they spoke to friends of his wife, they learned she had confided a plan to put an end to the family's poverty and misery. She had poisoned herself, her mother, and the five children.[126]

In a rural Florida town in 1988, a neighborly dispute escalated into a murder that took years to solve. Peggy Carr, and six other family members, were all poisoned with thallium, but only Peggy died. Unopened cola bottles were found to be tampered with and contained thallium. Eventually, their neighbor, George Trepal, who had spent time in prison for illegally making amphetamines, was arrested. In his home were found traces of thallium, the Agatha Christie novel *The Pale Horse*, about murders committed with thallium, as well as a machine to recap soda bottles. Trepal was convicted for the murder of Peggy Carr and sentenced to death.[127] In 2011 a NJ chemist poisoned her husband with thallium to avoid facing their impending divorce. She was sentenced to life in prison.[128]

Dr. Pasquale had more news. Peter's grandmother's death investigation was being reopened, and an order was issued in October 2021 to exhume her body for examination and testing. It took until April 2022 to get the toxicology results on the grandmother's remains. Per Dr. Pasquale, her thallium levels were "very, very high." The case was now a possible double homicide.

Late on the afternoon of April 26, 2022, after spending the day running around to help the CDC with their multistate adenovirus hepatitis investigation, I was staring at my computer screen catching up on emails when an arm thrust an envelope over my cubicle wall accompanied by the words, "The courier said it is important." Most of my snail mail is either drug advertisements or American Medical Association (AMA) membership solicitations and both land in the recycle bin unopened. The large manilla envelope was from the OCME and contained a copy of the heavy metal report on Peter. In addition to the elevated thallium level in his blood, thallium was found in the urine at greater than 1,000,000 µ/L and in the thigh wound at 1000 µ/L. Also found in the thigh wound was lead at 1200 µ/L and antimony at 1.4 µ/L. In Peter's urine, there was lead at 10 µ/L and barium at 8.5 µ/L. Trace levels of arsenic and mercury were also detected. Dr. Pasquale thought the other elements were consistent with background levels. I wasn't so sure and was especially intrigued by the lead found in the wound. Perhaps the proportion of each element found in the wound was a clue? Like how the chemical composition of an explosive can point to its origin. What products contained both thallium and lead?

I asked my brother, the one who broke his arm pretending he had a broken leg. He's an organic chemist but knows a lot about catalysts, which are often metals. He couldn't think of anything commercially available that contained both thallium and lead. I had some suspicions and turned to the internet to answer where lead and thallium and lead are found together. The searches turned up very little. So, I asked ChatGPT4[129] where lead and thallium are found together. The reply was in sulfide ore, other mineral, and volcanic deposits. I rephrased my question, where are lead and thallium found together in commercial products? This time the answer included batteries, alloys, electronics, industrial catalysts,pigments and dyes. I then asked what trace elements are in thallium-containing rat poisons. This time the answer was more informative. Trace elements that can be found in thallium-containing rat poisons include lead, cadmium, arsenic, mercury, and antimony.

The lethal dose of thallium, in the form of rat poison, for a three-year-old is about 150 mg or one-quarter of a teaspoon. Since the compound dissolves easily in water and is colorless, odorless, and tasteless, it would not be detected by the victim. Whoever may have killed Peter had access to him while in the hospital and may have sought to ensure his demise by additionally injecting him with the poison. That a parent could kill their child is inconceivable, but Peter's parents were possible suspects as they had the necessary access. And what about Peter's grandmother? An accidental exposure to thallium was conceivable but with Peter's death and his physical and laboratory findings, the grandmother's death was undeniably suspicious. What was the motive to kill her? Was it a practice run? Where would the assailant obtain thallium-based rat poisoning? Was it found in the storeroom of an old apartment building? The sale of thallium-based anything was banned in the United States fifty years ago, so that seems unlikely. What about importing from another country where it is legal? That would be risky as it would leave a paper trail. But what about the US black market?

In April 2022 it seemed as if NYPD was close to making an arrest, however, as of August 2024 no arrest has been made. I am not privy to the police investigation files, but search warrants were likely issued for the parents' residences to search for thallium. Since no charges have been filed, it stands to reason those searches turned up nothing. I don't think the case has been closed, and while the motive remains elusive, justice for Peter and his grandmother remain unfulfilled.

CHAPTER 16

Did the Commissioner Diddle While Rectums Burned?

I was convinced that COVID-19 would stand as the department and the City's biggest public health failure during my tenure, but I was about to be proven wrong. We could do worse. Monkeypox, or as it is now known mpox, had been a curious tropical disease but of little consequence in the United States. It was first identified in lab monkeys in 1958, and the first human case occurred in the Democratic Republic of Congo in 1970. It causes a disease that mimics smallpox, only less deadly. The illness begins with fever, headache, and fatigue before the rash appears and evolves through stages of flat red disks to pustules to crusting over.

Before 2003, Western Countries had little experience with the disease. In April 2003, an exotic pet dealer from Texas imported 600 small mammals from Ghana. Some were shipped to a distributor in Illinois where they were housed in cages adjacent to native prairie dogs, also to be sold as pets. Among the species imported that later tested positive for mpox were dormice, pouched rats, and rope squirrels, but it was the prairie dogs that fueled the outbreak. Forty-seven cases occurred in six midwestern states. All of the cases were attributed to contact with infected animals and none to either human skin-to-skin or person-to-person contact.[130] While mpox fatalities have been reported, mostly in African children, none of the outbreak cases died. Necropsy and testing of deceased prairie dogs identified viral replication in lung mucosal and tongue cells.[131] Pox transmission was believed to occur predominantly through an animal bite or contact with the rash, but transmission through animal respiratory secretions was not ruled out.

Former NYC police officer Eric Adams ran for mayor in 2021 as de Blasio served the limit of two terms. Adams won and created search committees to help him identify candidates to fill cabinet posts. One lead of the search committee for health commissioner was Ashwin Vasan, who was the CEO of Fountain House, a mental health nonprofit community organization. After a few weeks, a short period for identifying, interviewing, and vetting candidates for such an important position, Vasan got selected to be the next health commissioner. Vasan worked at the health department from 2016 to 2019, in a role for which his supervisors felt the need to have him take management coaching. Former female coworkers spoke anonymously with *Politico* reporter Amanda Eisenberg in 2022, and shared that they felt Vasan was "curt," "dismissive," and created a "toxic environment."[132] Vasan resigned in 2019 and didn't return to the workforce, according to the documents reviewed by *Politico*, for seven months, although he listed no periods of unemployment greater than four months on his paperwork to become health commissioner. He assumed the role of health commissioner in March 2022.

It was May 18, the D✪Ds were dealing with another surge of COVID-19 and I was tasked to investigate worrisome cases of suspected adenovirus hepatitis in children when Scott

Harper shared reports of mpox cases seemingly imported into several European Countries. The European Centre for Disease Prevention and Control (ECDC) issued a news release on May 19, 2022, reporting the first case was found in England on May 7 in a person who had traveled to Nigeria.[133] It was followed by six others with no contact with the first or travel to an endemic country. The last four were known to be MSM. Meanwhile, on the Iberian Peninsula, there were five confirmed mpox cases in MSM; over twenty suspect cases in Portugal, all in young men; and seven confirmed, and twenty-two suspect cases in Spain, all in men and many with a link to a sauna. A connection to attendance at Gay Pride events was also made, including the Maspalomas Gay Pride, which was held from May 5–15, 2022, in Spain. Very quickly mpox cases were recognized in the United States, Sweden, Italy, Belgium, Canada, Australia, France, Germany, the Netherlands, and Israel all by May 21. A reminder of just how far and fast disease can travel.

It was evident from the outset to practicing infectious disease epidemiologists that something new was occurring with mpox, specifically that it was likely being transmitted sexually. The major findings from patients were anogenital rashes. However, the initial public messaging emphasized that anyone can get mpox. While true, everyone wasn't getting mpox. Sexually active MSM were getting mpox. Mpox wasn't behaving like COVID-19. The messaging was analogous to saying anyone could get decompression sickness, an illness restricted to deep-sea divers. Or that anyone could get black lung disease, an illness of coal miners. It reminded me of a Seinfeld episode where Jerry and George are mistaken for a gay couple. Jerry proclaims, "We're not gay," and to distance themselves from homophobia quickly adds, "Not that there's anything wrong with that." The ensuing pressure to avoid stigmatization would paralyze public health into muddled prevention messaging and over-reliance on a limited supply of an imperfect vaccine.

The same day as the ECDC story appeared the first mpox case was diagnosed in NYC. Over the next four weeks the pandemic moved slowly, averaging about one case per day in the city. It was an opportunity to intervene. What puzzled me from the beginning of the pandemic was the reluctance by the CDC, and others, to accept that mpox was being sexually transmitted. This devolved into an esoteric wrestling match as to whether it was technically a sexually transmitted disease or was being transmitted during sexual encounters. Some claimed that mpox couldn't be classified as an STI because it's known to be transmitted skin-to-skin. But syphilis and herpes are transmitted skin-to-skin, and they are classified as STIs. Others said it can't be classified as a sexually transmitted disease until a live virus is found in semen. I did not doubt that mpox would be found in semen. Perhaps even in people before or without symptoms. That's because there were precedents, most recently with the Zika virus. The number of cases of proctitis where the sex partner had no genital rash also suggested semen was a source. But such studies take time, and when has public health allowed a lack of perfect knowledge to stop prevention interventions? Others claimed that the route of the majority of transmission determines whether a disease is an STI. Well, in this outbreak, sex was the overwhelming route of transmission. I found the STI-or-no argument pointless and unhelpful. Diseases change, a lesson we should have already learned. Regardless, public health messages failed to alert MSM about their risk.

Our practice had been that messages were crafted to the medical community by subject matter experts in a health alert (HAN).

HANs were then shared with the press office staffers who then crafted messages for the media and public. Before a press release was sent out, it was reviewed by subject matter experts to ensure the translation of science to lay terminology was clear and accurate. Under Commissioner Vasan, HANs underwent prodigious review while press releases did not reach the eyes of subject matter experts. Here's the mpox press release from June 13, 2022:

> *New Yorkers should take some steps to have a safe and joyous Pride month. To date, presumptive monkeypox cases have been identified in New York City and there is suspected community transmission occurring in the United States. The monkeypox virus is most often spread through direct contact with a rash or sores of someone who has the virus. It can also spread through contact with clothing, bedding, and other items used by a person with monkeypox, or from respiratory droplets that can be passed in close contact. Anyone can get and spread monkeypox, but currently, most cases are among gay, bisexual, and other men who have sex with men. People who have a new or unexpected rash or sores (which may look like pimples or blisters) anywhere on their body should seek care.[134]*

The press release alludes to community transmission in the United States, but the wording suggests not in NYC. The emphasis of the risk message is on contact with infected individuals and bedding, an egregious overstatement. Included was the oft used and highly misleading phrase, "Anyone can get and spread monkeypox." Cases were nearly exclusively in MSM, but there was no mention of sex as the major route of transmission in the press release.

The department wasn't the only source of muddled messaging.

There's an expectation in science and public health that subject matter experts are current on the published literature. If not individually, then collectively. Therefore, the CDC should have been aware of several articles published on mpox that raised the possibility of sexual transmission. Dimie Ogoina and coauthors published in PLOS ONE in 2019 details of a mpox outbreak that occurred in Nigeria. In their discussion is this paragraph:

> *It is noteworthy that a substantial number of our cases who were young adults in their reproductive age presented with genital ulcers, as well as concomitant syphilis and HIV infection. Although the role of sexual transmission of human monkeypox is not established, sexual transmission is plausible in some of these patients through close skin-to-skin contact during sexual intercourse or by transmission via genital secretions.*[135]

The sexual histories of persons in the Nigerian outbreak were explored and revealed high-risk activities, such as multiple concurrent sexual partners and transactional sex. All persons identified as heterosexual, but of twenty-one patients from the initial outbreak, seventeen were males. It is important to note that Nigeria criminalizes same-sex activity and marriage.

The CDC's initial message was distributed on May 20, 2022. The second sentence of their health alert described in detail what the rash of mpox looked like, that it is "firm, well circumscribed, deep-seated, and umbilicated."[136] No mention was made of the anogenital locations of the rash until some 250 words later. Near the end of the summary, is the risk factor, "A man who regularly has close or intimate in-person contact with other men, including those met through an online website, digital application (app), or at a bar or party." The words left out of the risk were, "for sex." Finally, was this sentence, "Lesions may be disseminated or located on the genital or perianal area alone."

Well-known and respected risk communication expert, Peter Sandman, who had provided multiple training sessions to the department, shared his thoughts with a reporter from the University of Minnesota's Center for Infectious Disease Research and Policy (CIDRAP). Sandman was sensitive to the issue of stigma but clearly placed protecting health above concerns over stigma. Furthermore, he challenged that public health officials were not actually seeking to prevent stigma but protecting themselves from being criticized for stoking stigma.[137] On his website Sandman wrote: "It's horrifying when public health officials (or reporters covering public health issues) pussyfoot around stigma concerns in ways that fail to give people the information they need to make decent decisions about their own health."[138]

We were averaging two to four new cases per day and the stories we were hearing and photographs we were seeing were different from what was known about mpox. The lesions were smaller, less obviously pustular, and the locations were unusual: perianal, penile, rectal, and oral. All the NYC cases were in MSM. As the City was preparing to distribute a limited supply of vaccine— JYNNEOS, a vaccinia-based product for both smallpox and mpox—I sent the following sequence of emails to several department colleagues.

From: Don Weiss
Sent: Thursday, June 16, 2022 8:50 A.M.
To: Redacted
Subject: RE: HCW PeP vaccine for positive MP case

At the risk of being blasted into politically incorrect oblivion, when this has nothing to do with politics, wouldn't refraining from anonymous sex for two incubation periods end the outbreak at a much lower cost and energy?

Have there been any prevention messages to the MSM community?

From: Don Weiss <Dweiss@health.nyc.gov>
Sent: Thursday, June 16, 2022 1:25 P.M.
To: Redacted
Subject: RE: CDC updated the clinical FAQ to address condom use after finishing isolation

Well, I am also wondering why no prevention message has gone out, as I've said, this outbreak could be stopped if the community took a few (temporary) steps to place a moratorium on anonymous sex.

When there's contaminated lettuce, people stop buying and eating.

From: Don Weiss
Sent: Thursday, June 16, 2022 4:52 PM
To: Redacted
Subject: sad prediction

MPX will become an endemic STI in NYC, taking its place alongside gonorrhea, chlamydia, syphilis and herpes. Soon we will start to see cases in women, then among non-MSM and not long after that we will have our first congenital infection. It will happen on our watch. We cannot vaccinate our way out of this, nor can we isolate our way out of this. The only way out is to abstain. I know I sound like a bible thumping preacher, but this is the exposure we need to PREVENT. We don't have much time to intervene and it may already be too late.

Others were thinking along similar lines. On June 17, 2022, an associate professor of Infectious Diseases at a prestigious university alerted us to new mpox messaging posted on the CDC's website. He asked the following question in an email which was forwarded to me:

> *Can anyone explain the CDC safer sex for monkeypox advice (link and excerpt below)? Particularly the part about sex with clothes on. There are lurid headlines coming out. It does mention that best way to prevent spread is abstinence, but the alternative strategies listed do not appear evidence based.*

> *If you or your partner have (or think you might have) monkeypox and you decide to have sex, consider the following to reduce the chance of spreading the virus:*
> *–Have virtual sex with no in-person contact.*
> *–Masturbate together at a distance of at least 6 feet, without touching each other and without touching any rash or sores.*
> **–Consider having sex with your clothes on or covering areas where rash or sores are present, reducing as much skin-to-skin contact as possible.**
> *–Avoid kissing.*
> *–Remember to wash your hands, fetish gear, sex toys and any fabrics (bedding, towels, clothing) after having sex*
> *–Limit your number of partners to avoid opportunities for monkeypox to spread.*

As much as the message was infuriating, I was heartened to hear that we weren't the only ones struggling to clear up the muddled messaging. One could argue that the avoidance-of-risky-sex message was included. But that's not how humans behave. Given the choice of several, presumably equally effective options, people pick the path of least resistance. What's more, the severity of illnesses and consequences were not clearly shared. Specifically, that mpox proctitis can be a week-long, agonizing illness. I sent yet another email.

From: Don Weiss
Sent: Wednesday, June 22, 2022 8:18 AM
To: Redacted
Cc: Redacted
Subject: RE: team assignments

This disease is entirely preventable had we the courage to send out prevention messages. I understand the reluctance to warn people to refrain from anonymous sex, yet harm reduction has not made an appearance. We seem paralyzed by the fear of stigmatizing this disease while we totally ignore the epidemiology. If we had an outbreak associated with bowling, would we not warn people to stop bowling?

ICS was activated on June 21, 2022, at about the same time my ex-girlfriend, Lindsay, was dying of ovarian cancer. She was a nurse who had done STI partner notification, was a contra dancer, and universally loved by all who knew her. Lindsay's close friend had survived the same disease, but she wouldn't be so lucky. We had met in St. Louis, but she was living in Maine. I wanted to visit, but she asked that I not.

ICS conference calls were held every Tuesday and Thursday. A few months earlier, I had gotten myself ejected from COVID-19 ICS duties because I had written in an email—many emails, but one got forwarded—that I believed de Blasio's replacement for health commissioner, Dr. Dave Chokshi, was a puppet commissioner. Chokshi had told Marci that he was sent to the department to stop leaks to the media. In my reading of his credentials, he had negligible public health experience and hadn't managed anything near the size of the department. I suspected that he'd do whatever the mayor asked, having been told to be distrustful of the D⊗Ds, while having little knowledge himself of applied public health.

Celia Quinn, Demetre's replacement, was the person who admonished and banished me. I didn't mind being sent to the doghouse as my day-to-day work hadn't changed except that I had fewer meetings and encounters with newly hired unqualified staff. But like Michael Corleone in *The Godfather*, just when I thought I was out, they pulled me back in. I was told that I would again be co-lead of the SurvEpi branch for the mpox response. Since the other co-lead hadn't yet played any role yet in the mpox pandemic, the job mostly fell to me.

At 2 p.m. we had the first ICS call, and I learned there was going to be a vaccine clinic at the Chelsea STI Center opening on Thursday, June 23. The vaccine clinic was to run for four days and there were 1,000 available doses. The CDC had told us that there were 64,000 doses of JYNNEOS vaccine in the national stockpile, and for phase one, they were releasing 56,000 doses to be distributed to the sites with the most cases. More vaccines would be made available from manufacturers in the coming weeks. Some doses were in storage, and the rest had to be made—perhaps 500,000 additional doses, but the sum of 7 million was also mentioned.

No timeline was given. However, the CDC also admitted that there wasn't enough vaccine to go around. The number of MSM in NYC in 2022 was estimated to be somewhere between 200,000 to 400,000. I voiced my concern during the ICS meeting that our vaccine plan was not well thought out, that there would be tremendous demand, and that it could create a very chaotic situation. I was ignored. There had to be a problem with the CDC's math in calculating NYC's allotment of vaccine, but the department did nothing to remedy it. We just sailed forward straight into an iceberg.

The vaccine rollout went beyond mere chaos. With so few doses the intent was to prioritize persons who had an exposure to a mpox patient. The demand was as expected, overwhelming. Lines were long and tempers short. Many people were turned away. The Chelsea Center was forced to close after the clinic operations manager was threatened with violence. The appointment scheduler crashed after what the department said was an unexpected level of traffic. There was fear and panic, despite the commissioner's blithe pleas otherwise. Here's what Vasan had to say:

> This is not a time for anxiety and panic. This is a time for preparation and I think that's what we're trying to show. That we're standing up and stepping up for the community by offering up this first-in-the-country resource.[139]

Time for preparation? We were unprepared. And the plug about being first? Empty and egotistical. The department had failed to communicate sufficiently about mpox and failed to anticipate the demand and plan appropriately. We should have demanded that the CDC release more vaccine to NYC. We had the data to justify. One X/Twitter user gave us an "F" for our vaccine rollout.

Like COVID-19, the SurvEpi branch was swamped when it was tasked to arrange a rotating group of medical epidemiologists to triage calls from providers reporting suspected cases and to arrange testing. Like COVID-19, testing for mpox in the first phase of the pandemic was only available at public health labs and the CDC. Our lab could do an orthopox screening test, but the CDC had to confirm mpox. We asked ICS for additional staff, and they responded by sending emails to staff already mobilized.

We were soon triaging sixty to eighty calls a day from providers looking for testing for their patients. But our lab could only test twenty specimens a day, so we were again asked to be gatekeepers. Even so, we accepted more each day than could be tested and the lab got backed up. Similar to the ECDC report, the patients were men who had rash eruptions in the perianal and genital areas, people with penile lesions, and those who claimed their partners didn't have a rash. Almost every case we sent for testing came back positive. The outbreak was taking off.

The calls we received from medical providers were disturbing in other regards. One patient had a solitary ulcer on his lip that arose three days after his last sexual contact. He neither had a prodrome nor a disseminated rash, no fever, muscle aches, or headache. The incubation period was incredibly short, and he tested positive. The virus was behaving in an entirely new way. Heart wrenching stories about painful proctitis were difficult to hear. Excruciating pain, along with inflammation and ulceration of the anal canal, turned the mundane bodily function of defecation into a Marquis de Sade torture. One physician described normal appearing perianal skin, but when he viewed the rectum through an anoscope he saw ulcerated and bleeding mucosa. The patients pleaded for treatment but there was only one medication, tecovirimat, known as TPOXX. The drug didn't have FDA approval and was only dispensed under an investigational new drug protocol. So, getting it for a patient required the physician to jump through hoops, while underwater, carrying a hundred- pound sack of rocks. This meant reams of paperwork and miles of red tape. Many physicians didn't have the wherewithal or time. D✪D Dr. Ellen Lee took it upon herself to get as many patients as she could TPOXX.

The first time I recall stigma being raised as a concern was in mid-June on a conference call with the CDC, state and local public health officials, and community-based organizations. Demetre Daskalakis, who after leaving the department mid-COVID-19, had become the CDC director of HIV/AIDS prevention, did most of the talking, and his message, once I stripped away the double-speak and cliché, was that mpox is not a gay disease. No one raised a sex moratorium or some form of abstinence as an option for prevention. No safe sex messages such as monogamy, avoiding anonymous partners, and sex parties. Despite the gravity of the situation, it remained a taboo subject. The impression I was left with was that gay sex is like oxygen; you can't deprive it. The call ended with a chorus of back slapping. Everyone was fabulous, everyone learned, it was wonderful. Yet calls from the NYC medical community kept coming. Many patients reported that they didn't know what to look for, another failure of the department's communication strategy. I had a foreboding premonition of what was to come.

For context, ICS pulls staff from throughout the department and places them into emergency response groups (ERG). There is an incident commander who is in charge and runs the meeting. The ERGs include planning, logistics, information technology, finance, community engagement, clinical operations, and environmental operations. SurvEpi is in the clinical operations section along with the laboratory, provider communications, and vaccine management, among others. Other members include the public information officer, legal officer, equity officer, and safety officer. Typically, representatives from the commissioner's office attend and monitor the discussions and decisions. In early July, during two ICS calls, I tried again to insert logic into our messaging.

I told the group that vaccination alone was not going to be enough to stop transmission, that we needed to advise MSM to alter their sexual practices. We weren't doing enough through public messaging to alert MSM to the symptoms and risk factors, specifically what the epidemiology was telling us about how it was being transmitted. It wasn't being transmitted via linens, or casual skin-to-skin contact, or even through respiratory droplets. It was sex, specifically, oral and anal sex. It was also likely that live virus would be found in semen and that infected persons were likely infectious before symptoms appeared or had no discernible symptoms at all. I shared with ICS the painful descriptions of mpox proctitis and that treatment was not very accessible. I stressed again that we had to do a better job at prevention. Whereas we had dozens of public service announcements on COVID-19, there wasn't one yet on mpox.

The first time I raised these issues there was no response. Celia Quinn, the incident commander, just moved on. The second time there was a brief exchange where Quinn, and the public information officer, Maura Kennelly, informed me that they were working through community partners to get the message out. I wanted to hear more. What subject matter experts were in those meetings? Who were the CBOs? What were the messages? How were they being communicated? Nothing more was shared, and I felt

---

gaslighted, but I had done what I could to alert leadership.

Triaging calls, arranging testing, and getting patients TPOXX felt like attempting to squeeze a dirigible through the eye of a needle. The calls from medical providers were overwhelming. The PHL was backlogged. The D✚Ds were stressed, hungry, tired, and in need of bathroom breaks. Staff who survived the threat and stress of COVID-19, were again being put through a meat grinder and I doubted many would return for thirds. The most disheartening aspect was that mpox was preventable. It should've been common knowledge among the gay community that mpox is circulating, yet we repeatedly heard about men having multiple unprotected sexual encounters who hadn't heard the message. Why wasn't the mayor, commissioner, and other civic leaders telling the community what I felt they needed to know to protect themselves? Mpox proctitis and pharyngitis were not pleasant and should be reason enough to abstain from risky sex. We seemed to be waiting for the entire MSM population to become immune, either from infection or vaccination, and we had many more weeks to go.

Preeti Pathela, the SurvEpi co leader, emailed the incident commander to inform her that we needed more staff to keep up. She also pushed the argument for better communication. Preeti was a STI epidemiologist, so she knew the terrain. She pointed out that public awareness about transmission and risk was lacking and that SurvEpi should be part of the brainstorming process. She also pointed out our website's deficiencies. Overall, it was too hard to find information and the MSM messages were not prominent enough. Preeti succeeded in getting a call scheduled, but no sooner had we begun the conversation, that Celia Quinn announced that she didn't know what the call was about and said she was prepared to discuss how we could handle the surge in calls and cases. The response plan for the mpox typhoon was to continue to rely on mopping up the floor instead of closing the windows.

The media continued publishing quotes from public health pundits that mpox was not a sexually transmitted disease. While at the gym on Sunday, July 10, an MSNBC medical reporter said mpox wasn't a sexually transmitted disease and emphasized skin-to-skin contact. She then went on to say that people who think they might have been exposed should go to their doctor and get tested. Wrong advice. Mpox wasn't like COVID-19, there was no testing for exposure. Previously she claimed that vaccine was prevention *and* treatment while holding off on mentioning the risk to MSM until the last seconds of the interview.[140] The department wasn't speaking up, so the void was being filled with misinformation.

None of the media spokespeople had any firsthand knowledge of the situation, but they were only too happy to have a microphone to share their opinions. Mary Bassett was now the New York State health commissioner. She too, said mpox wasn't an STI. But days later, on a July 11 town hall video conference call with health department staff, she reversed this. Whether or not mpox was an STI was an academic argument, but I felt that saying definitively that it wasn't was a disservice to the MSM community. The message being that if mpox was not a STI, then there was no need to alter behavior. On the town hall call, which Commissioner Vasan also participated in, they said all the right things. That MSM should avoid sex at clubs, parties, and other mass gatherings. But it was to the wrong audience.

Cases counts kept rising. Providers were confused and the HAN, which would provide the missing information, was still under review because what was inserted didn't align with the recent press release or website—neither of which we were asked to provide input. The press release continued to emphasize that anyone can get monkeypox. On the website was the familiar refrain that coming in contact with bedding or other items during or after intimate activity. They couldn't even write the word sex, cloaking the advice in vague language. Sexual activity was the risk, not the bedding! This message was tantamount to advising people who were just hit by a bus and lying in the street to take care that people leaving the bus didn't trample them on their way out.

Patients' experiences continued to highlight the absence of communication with medical providers and the population at risk. One patient texted about his experience at a NYC hospital, stating he was placed in an isolation room for hours and was examined through the window. Doctors then took pictures through the window making him feel like a zoo animal. The patient bemoaned the misinformation and lack of preparedness and was planning to speak out about how the department was handling the crisis.

A person who had already tested positive for mpox developed proctitis and sought care. He confided to the provider that he had attended the Nubian Dukes sex party in Manhattan in late June that was attended by an estimated 100 people. He reported that he had anal receptive sex with approximately fifty people. The provider wasn't interested in the information.

Another patient voiced a new concern, that MSM will think that a single dose of vaccine will rescue them when two doses are required, and the vaccine was never studied to provide mucosal immunity or protect against sexual transmission. He was prescient as a man in his mid-20s had received a vaccine dose in the first week of July. He then had four, new male sex partners. On July 10, he had a fever and the eruption of a red fluid-filled tender rash on his face. He tested positive for mpox.

Preeti's demeanor was typically measured and cool-headed,

but even she was exasperated. She wrote, "We have to find a way to get information out about these types of risk. We're doing people a disservice by downplaying the facts." I believed it was only a matter of time before science would document the virus in semen, both before rash onset and in those who never have symptoms. The great tragedy of mpox is that government and public health leaders have monumentally failed to act and are guilty of ignoring the evidence and the experience of their staff.

Standard public health communication practice involves the determination of risk factors and then providing the population with the information they need to protect themselves. When the 1992 outbreak of *E.coli* O157:H7 was traced to hamburgers from one specific fast-food chain the message to the public was clear: Avoid Jack in the Box until further notice, which was only until the tainted beef was removed from circulation. Whenever there's a contaminated food product, be it lettuce, strawberries, deli turkey meat, or oysters, the public is advised to avoid, return product, or dispose. Brand names are not withheld. When Canadian wildfires made the air unsafe for people with respiratory conditions to breathe, the message was to stay indoors. Did this message stigmatize asthmatics? There are endless examples—imported candy tainted with lead, cribs with unsafe slats, pacifiers able to choke infants, sharks near the shoreline, excessive heat conditions, and vehicles at risk of rollovers. The public is informed, dangerous products are recalled, action steps shared, and in some instances regulations enacted. Did public health hesitate over concerns of stigmatizing Jack in the Box? No, safety trumps all other concerns. Why was mpox different? Because the population at risk were gay men? Because of historical regrets? We had information about mpox risk and consequences. The job of public health is to tell people what we know, share prevention guidance, and allow people to make their own decisions—individually and as a community.

The death blow to public health credibility came late on Friday, July 15, 2022. It was a press release issued by the department. No one in SurvEpi was asked to review it. In it were these words:

> *In addition to vaccine, prevention measures offer pro-tection. These include avoiding close physical contact if sick, especially if there is a new or unexpected rash or sore. For those who choose to have sex while sick, it is best to avoid kissing and other face-to-face contact. Also, sores should be covered with clothing or sealed bandages. This may help reduce — but not eliminate — the risk of transmission.*[141]

This press release recycled the embarrassing, month-old, unscientific, CDC messaging that was roundly criticized. It ignored the evidence collected by the department's own staff. The words about avoiding risky sexual intercourse, spoken by the health commissioner just four days earlier during the town hall conference call, seem to have been forgotten as soon as they left his mouth. And once again, the fear of being called out as a stig-matist outweighed honest, direct, disease preventing messaging.

I took to email to alert SurvEpi and other ICS colleagues:

From: Don Weiss
Sent: Friday, July 15, 2022 4:30 PM
To: redacted
Subject: FW: NYC HEALTH DEPARTMENT ON MONKEYPOX VACCINATION STRATEGY AND PRIORITIZATION OF FIRST DOSES

Did you see this press statement? Unbelievable. After all the rhetoric on the town hall from Vasan and Bassett this is the message in last paragraph below?

In addition to vaccine, prevention measures offer protection. These include avoiding close physical contact if sick, especially if there is a new or unexpected rash or sore. For those who choose to have sex while sick, it is best to avoid kissing and other face-to-face contact. Also, sores should be covered with clothing or sealed bandages. This may help reduce — but not eliminate — the risk of transmission

Message should be:

If you wish to avoid monkeypox, DON'T HAVE SEX, most importantly, not anonymous/multiple partner sex.

From: Don Weiss
Sent: Friday, July 15, 2022 4:40 PM
To: redacted
Subject: RE: NYC HEALTH DEPARTMENT ON MONKEYPOX VACCINATION STRATEGY AND PRIORITIZATION OF FIRST DOSES

The virus is very likely in semen and saliva. I also think a person without symptoms can pass the virus, another fact that will take time to prove. If we wish to prevent transmission we should message these likelihoods. It is no different than other STIs- the risk is from having sex with a non-monogamous partner.

I received a flurry of replies:

"It's mind boggling. Cover sores with clothing or bandages? Cover penile and peri-anal lesions? Avoid kissing? Face-to-face contact? Seriously?"

"Do you know if there is any vetting of press releases by knowledgeable medical personnel here at DOHMH? Some of the crap that comes out is unfathomable."

"WOAH!!!"

"Wowza!!!"

"Making it crystal clear here that I AGREE!! Very very problematic. And dangerous."

"Tom Frieden, Mary Bassett, and Sue Blank... never would have tolerated how we have refused to speak frankly while a sexually transmitted disease rampaged through LGBT communities... silence=complicity."

"Why are we putting ourselves in the position to do damage control? Damage that has come from within, despite our group repeatedly insisting that the messages need to be clear, direct, and unafraid? It's terrible for the community and making our jobs so much harder."

"Definitely don't know of anyone with an epi brain here who was asked to review this!"

Those colleagues were fellow DODs and epidemiologists from bureaus within the Division of Disease Control. Persons with ten to twenty years of hands-on, public health experience in STIs and HIV. It was good to know we were aligned, but our voices, individually and collectively, had been, in my opinion, and would likely continue to be ignored. By the time we all returned to work the following Monday, there'd be more than 500 mpox cases. NYC was the epicenter of the outbreak. Something needed to be done. As I rode home, I saw only one option. There was a reporter at *The New York Times* who continued to seek me out for information. I had thus far refused. Prior to COVID-19 and mpox, the higher-level administrators at the department had been knowledgeable, experienced, and reasonable people. They listened to Marci Layton and the D❂Ds and changed course when appropriate. Many, including Marci, had moved on and were largely replaced by novices, most of whom didn't see the need or value in soliciting input from subject matter experts. They seemed to me to behave like children allowed to play with loaded guns, too naive to recognize the danger. But they were adults. I emailed Joseph Goldstein at *The New York Times* and told him I was ready to talk. On the record.

Joseph Goldstein's article was published in *The New York Times* online on July 18, 2024, and in print the next day. The message to the gay community was that mpox was spreading through sex and prevention required their collective action, to temporarily reduce the number of sex partners.[142] The rebuttal from the department was the anti-stigma and sex-positive rhetoric. Three days after the article was published, I was summoned to a meeting with human resources where I was informed that I was being transferred to the Bureau of Maternal and Child Health. The justification was called a realignment. Amid a burgeoning pandemic, when the department was scrambling to find experienced staff to support the response, an experienced infectious disease epidemiologist was being transferred to a bureau that had neither asked for nor sought help in the form of a job posting. It was tantamount to transferring a firefighter from the frontline of a wildfire back to the station to open the mail. My words apparently embarrassed the commissioner, and his response was like a Banana Republic dictator by jailing the opposition leader to silence dissent.

Speaking to the media without authorization was an unwritten rule. Firing me would have been protracted and difficult. I wasn't called to meet with the commissioner or supervisors to discuss my actions. Vasan's response provoked a cartoon image to form in my mind. I can't draw, but I envisioned a poignant *New Yorker* cartoon. In it, Vasan is wearing a toga and laurel leaf crown. He's standing on a hill, fiddle in hand, overlooking the city which is in ruins. Men are running to and fro, panicked and in pain, arms thrust backward as fire blazes from their backsides. I am not making light of the situation, only what I perceive to be the dumb and self-serving decisions and responses by the health commissioner. The pain MSM experienced was real, as was our empathy, and desire to intervene.

Following the publication of *The New York Times* article, Commissioner Vasan did interviews to defend his position. To CNN reporter Naomi Thomas, he said on July 21, "The best thing for the city is getting shots in arms as quickly as possible… and give them the information to tell them how monkeypox is transmitted."[143] Not quite. According to a study published in *The New England Journal of Medicine*, the two-dose regimen of the JYNNEOS vaccine was 66% effective, and a single dose was only 36% effective.[144] Only one-third of recipients received two doses according to data published on the department website on November 17, 2022. Additionally, the vaccine takes several weeks before it becomes effective, and a person won't know if they are protected if exposed during a sexual encounter. Relying on vaccination, and avoiding correct messaging was, in my twenty-two years of experience, the wrong strategies.

And what about the line, "give them the information to tell them how monkeypox is transmitted"? Giving the community the information we knew on how mpox was being transmitted, and precisely how the illness was manifesting, was what we were imploring the department to release, but instead the department said to "cover your sores." The second mpox HAN, which updated providers on the epidemiology and clinical manifestations of mpox, was begun in late June, but was delayed by the commissioner's office until July 18.

From Vasan's interview with CNN also came this:

> *Gay men, men who have sex with men, and the LGBTQ community writ large, have had their sexual practices and behaviors dissected and prescribed and permitted mostly by heterosexual people … coming out of the HIV movement, [that's] really, really damaging and stigmatizing and discriminatory.*[145]

Vasan was an infant during the HIV movement and had been on the job for all of four months in July 2022. Typical of my perception of megalomaniacs, he seemed to believe he knew best. One benefit of speaking out to *The New York Times* was that it provoked discussion and allowed people to educate themselves. Many members of the gay community didn't agree with Vasan. Ben Ryan, a journalist with interest in public health wrote in *The Washington Post:*

> *Many officials have shied away from clear statements about how the public can best protect themselves. Crucially, they have often failed to communicate emerging scientific theories that if men avoid anal sex — or perhaps use a condom during intercourse — they might at least limit some of the most devastating monkeypox symptoms, including severe proctitis.*[146]

And…

> *This reluctance is driven by an entrenched belief that telling gay men to alter our sexual practices is intrinsically homophobic or stigmatizing… this thinking also patronizes gay men as perennial adolescents… we deserve the government's best advice on how to protect ourselves now.*[147]

Mark King. activist and author, wrote in *POZ:*

> *Will there be stigma and judgments and homophobia? Of course. And we'll have to deal with that. But that doesn't mean we bury crucial facts in vague, evasive messaging. Monkeypox is a gay thing. That's the truth.*[148]

Jim Downs, a history professor at Gettysburg College who studies infectious diseases, shared his perspective early in the pandemic in an *Atlantic* article:

> *For me, the most relevant information about monkeypox comes not from the history of the 1920s or the '80s but from the social media testimony of patients who are now suffering excruciating symptoms….*
>
> *I am not calling for the government to shut down gay establishments, not even bathhouses. I would prefer that gay men made the decision to be careful of their own volition. But I would also hope that public officials would base their recommendations to gay men on current information about the monkeypox outbreak.*[149]

I received many comments posted to my blog, Doctor With a Badge:[150]

"I admire your forthrightness in The New York Times. As a gay man who survived the AIDS epidemic, I pretty much reached the conclusion that abstinence, at least in the short term, was the most practical way to avoid monkeypox infection.

In another comment an infectious disease physician and HIV care provider had similar concerns about the messaging and agreed that advising gay men to limit their number of partners was an appropriate message. Another commenter thanked me for speaking up, stating, "The only stigma that I feel is being a gay man who disagrees with how 'activists' have tried to gaslight public health."

Peter Sandman wasn't the only person who placed the facts over the fear of stigmatization. Articles appeared in *POZ, The Atlantic, The Guardian,* and *The Daily Signal* arguing that giving MSM the facts they needed to protect themselves was not stigmatizing, but the role of public health officials and politicians. Muddling the messaging was, to me, the equivalent of dereliction of duty. The reluctance to speak truthfully about transmission was not to protect the gay community, but out of the fear of being canceled or labeled as homophobic. The lies of omission exposed countless people to harm that could've and should've been avoided.

Evidence has since come to light that not only is live virus present in saliva and semen, but it may also persist for months. A study published in *The British Medical Journal* in October of 2022 concluded that there was "considerable pre-symptomatic transmission, which was validated through linked patient level."[151] Despite the distribution of 150,000 doses of vaccine, mpox is still with us. In 2023 there were 171 mpox cases in NYC. During the first six months of 2024 there have been 264 cases. Mpox has become endemic in NYC. There is likely a significant quantity of immunity among the gay community, but over time, this will wane and the mpox epidemic could make a return.

It took until the late summer and fall of 2022 for the WHO, CDC, NYS, and NYC to change their messaging to concede that mpox was effectively an STI, and to revise their advice to MSM, that they should indeed avoid anonymous and multiple sex partners. It was far too late.

During an NPR interview on September 28, 2022, Demetre Daskalakis credited a CDC publication (and therefore himself) for the decline in cases, saying that MSM altered their behavior.[152] However, Demetre was, in my opinion, the chief architect of stigma-phobia and muddled messaging. As the White House's national monkeypox deputy coordinator, I suspect it may have been him who suggested or approved the wording that one could cover mpox sores or wear clothes, and still engage in sex. A warning for all of us: When there are no credible leaders, people will follow the charismatic, no matter how misguided they may be. And for those in power, when you care more about keeping your job than performing it, do the world a favor: quit.

The Future of Public Health

The foundation of human society is rules mutually agreed upon by its members. Some rules are codified as laws, such as theft and littering. Others are put forth by businesses, "no shoes, no shirt, no service." We've accepted that we must wait our turn on lines, can't urinate in public, must shower before entering the public pool, and have to pick up after our dogs. Many rules and laws are not strictly enforced, and we rely on each other to obey them so that we all can freely enjoy the benefits of modern society. Imagine if you can that your house is on fire. The fire department arrives and puts out the fire, saving your home from total destruction, but you object to how they did their job. You verbally and physically threaten them, picket outside their homes, and harass their children because the firefighters doused water on your belongings. Using social media, you enlist others to join you in your crusade and soon you elect a sympathizer to public office who seeks to curtail the fire department's powers. Sounds ridiculous, doesn't it?

Public health has operated in the background for decades, rarely coming to the public's consciousness. Sewer systems were built to remove waste from communities. Water treatment plants provide disease free water. Lead was removed from paint and gasoline to protect children from its harmful effects. Seat belts reduced automobile fatalities. Window guards, tobacco control, medication regulation, consumer product safety, food purity laws, the list goes on and on. Perhaps the single greatest innovation that has improved both the length and quality of life has been vaccinations. Diphtheria suffocated upwards of 15,000 Americans per year, most of them children, before the widespread use of vaccine. Polio killed and crippled, dooming some of its victims to a life in an iron lung machine. Smallpox was a major human scourge that is no more thanks to vaccine. Life expectancy has increased by twenty-five years, in a large part due to these and other public health innovations. Yet public health has been taken for granted.

COVID-19 was an unprecedented event. Unlike the 2009 pandemic of H1N1 influenza, there was no vaccine system in place nor available treatment when COVID-19 emerged and circled the globe. Decisions had to be made quickly with absent or imperfect data. Too often politicians, instead of engaging in healthy discussion with public health officials, believed they knew best. Mistakes were made and policies clung to either too long or not long enough. Public health officials did not get to set policy, and it is important to state that those decisions they were allowed to make were not based on personal gain nor with the intent to harm people physically, or economically. Yet blame fell on us. Many of my public health colleagues were fired or hounded out of office. Others took early retirement. Still others suffered through hostile environments made so by their elected leaders who stoked community outrage. Was wearing a mask while in indoor public spaces to protect others and your family such an egregious request? Compare this imposition to that of a loved one on a ventilator in the ICU. And consider how many of the people attacking public health would not have been born had their ancestors not been protected from disease, injury, and toxins by public health laws.

Public health has long faced uncertain funding. The responsibility of public health belongs to the states, which has resulted in wide disparities across the US with the common denominator of underfunding. The Federal Government, predominantly through the CDC, has tried to fill the gap but there has been a disconcerting pattern. When public health succeeds in reducing the burden of a health problem away goes the funding. Tuberculosis returned with a vengeance during the AIDS epidemic in part because funding dried up. Money flowed when West Nile virus emerged, then that money went away. After 9/11 there was an influx of money for preparedness but those funds gradually diminished until the next event, pandemic H1N1. So, it has gone with successive public health threats: Ebola, Zika virus, and now COVID-19. It has been fiscal Whac-A-Mole. Each round of funding was siloed, limiting how local public health jurisdictions could use the money to address their specific needs.

Following COVID-19, over twenty states enacted laws restricting public health powers or reallocating them to elected officials without the requisite expertise and experience to use the powers to protect their citizens. There is a lack of public trust created by politicians and a myriad of pundits and conspiracy theorists. Add to this no clear and respected voice, a depleted workforce, a leadership void, and a lack of reliable funding; the future of public health is at a crossroad. One thing we can be certain of is that threats to community health will continue to occur. Be they in the form of pandemics, war, or global warming induced weather events will be immaterial, if we are not prepared to face them. I think we all would agree that a society without the services of sanitation, fire, water, and police would not be a society at all. Public health needs to be a fully supported public work, like the aforementioned services of public safety.

After I spoke to the media about the health department's dysfunctional mpox messaging I was reassigned to the Bureau of Maternal and Child Health and sent to a satellite office, away from my former colleagues, and the health department administration. No reason was given, not that any would make sense. The commissioner's transfer of an experienced infectious disease epidemiologist during two pandemics to a program that hadn't asked for help felt purely punitive. My task was to make training slide sets for nurses who performed newborn home visits. I discovered that there were professionally made, and content accurate, videos available free online. My new bosses were unaware of this resource. Clearly, they were instructed to give me busy work in the hopes that I would resign. I doubt the slide sets I prepared have or ever will be used. Several months after the transfer I was made an offer I couldn't refuse. In 2018, I set a five-year exit plan from the health department. I volunteered at a summer basketball camp, performed free training with college players, and coached a seventh-grade team. The offer I couldn't refuse was to become an assistant coach for a university women's basketball team. I will also be teaching epidemiology to undergraduates, hopefully inspiring the next generation of D✪Ds.

On September 23, 2024, after two-and-half years on the job, Commissioner Vasan announced his resignation and that he would be leaving his post at the end of the year. The reason stated was to spend more time with family and he said the decision bore no relationship to the mayor's mounting legal troubles. Three days later, NYC Mayor Eric Adams, who had appointed Vasan, was indicted on federal corruption charges. It is alleged that Adams accepted money in quid pro quo deals with foreign agents. Mayor Adams has denied the charges or any wrongdoing. Less than a month later Vasan announced his immediate departure.[153] He has not been accused of any crimes. There may yet be more to the story.

ACKNOWLEDGMENTS

I am indebted to every D✪Ds who has worked for the Bureau of Communicable Disease. When I think back on my two decades as a D✪D what comes to mind aren't the frustrations, long hours, bureaucratic red tape, or arduous field visits. No, it's the humor, food, and celebrations. I recall how every holiday season staff spent their free time decorating a door with our Bureau's exploits. There was always a song with rewritten lyrics and a cannibalized melody. Penned by Beth, Paula or Alex and sung by a staff chorus. We even had a band, composed of D✪Ds, play live one season. For another door we built a jukebox that played recordings of our greatest hits. There were outbreak themed board games pinned to the door. Joel once dressed as Saint Nick and read the BCD version of Twas the Night Before Christmas. West Nile, anthrax, hepatitis, Zika virus all made appearances on doors with the goal of remembering, honoring, humanizing, and humoring the work that was often backbreaking. I've lost count of how many times we were selected as best overall door, but it was in the high teens. And while the door displays were extraordinary, they paled in comparison to the international smorgasbord that stretched from one end of the bureau to the other. Sally's vegetable lasagna, Asha's corn pudding, Joel's kugel, and my own slow simmered, barbecue brisket. There was always extra, and we invited staff from all over the department to be a D❂D for a day.

I fondly recall the energized and exciting faces of children we entertained on Take Our Children to Work days orchestrated by Stacey. Those junior D❂Ds conducted mock outbreak investigations, including restaurant inspections, sampling of cooling towers, simulated laboratory of testing mosquitoes and ticks plucked from a very realistic looking pseudo-forest created in our high-density files by Natasha. The priceless look of astonishment and discovery on Ellen's daughter's face as she pointed at a plastic rat emerging from a fake hole in the wall. Miranda using the "fogger" we built and filled with dry ice from her father's lab to simulate mosquito spraying. Chef Paula's comical yet abysmal food hygiene. There was a Baking Club, whose events were particularly delicious, especially Hilary's Pi Day (3.14). The Ample Hills Ice Cream Social. Wave Hill retreat. The Curmudgeon Club. The puns, poems, and book recommendations. What bittersweet farewell would be complete without Marci unfurling a several foot long blank scroll while saying she prepared, "a few words?" How when anyone was down on their luck or going through a rough stretch, there was always support in the form of cash, kindness, and casseroles.

Research assistance for *Disease Detectives* was provided by my nephew Scott Weiss and women's basketball players Brielle Guarente and Samatha Osorio. Special thanks to Drs. Marci Layton and Joel Ackelsberg for their support, recollections, and encouragement. Appreciation to Stephen Morse, who kindly read an early draft and penned the Forward, and to Brooke (another women's basketball player) for her artwork. Advance apologies to anyone I've omitted from the list of D❂Ds.

Abaynesh Minson, Alaina Stoute, Alan Dorsinville, Alexander Davidson, Alice Baptiste-Norville, Alice Yeung, Alison Levin-Rector, Alison Ridpath, Alison Whitney, Allison Piazza, Alyssa Chase Amanda Wahnich, Amber Whitcher, Ana Maria Fireteanu Andrea Econome, Andrea King, Andrea Lacayo, Andrea Seaborough, Angelica Bocour Ann Marie France, Ann Murray-Afordi, Ann Winters, Ann Winters, Ann Xing, Anna Smorodina, Anna Stachel, Anne Labowitz, Annie Fine, Antoinette Buckley, Anupa George, Asha Abdool, Ashley Cintron, Awilda Colon-Serrant, Ben Tsoi, Beth Fatato, Beth Maldin, Beth Nivin, Betty Ng, Bianca Malcolm, Bindy Crouch, Brianna Beaver-Timmons, Brooke Bregman, Bruce Gutelius, Bryan Cherry, Camille Aldolphe, Candacy Browne, Candice Clarke, Carl Jones, Carla Rodriguez, Carmen Roman, Carolina Alcala, Carolyn Coakes, CaSaundra Bush, Cassandra Harrison, Catharine Prussing, Catherine Addei-Maanu, Catherine Dentinger, Celia Deane Joe, Chantal Hall, Cheng Zhang, Chris Lee, Christopher Godfrey, Corinne Thompson, Dale McShine, Damon Duquaine, Dan Cimini, Dana Meranus, Dana Patrick, Daniel Calder, Daniel Chijioke, Daniel Krieger, Danielle Bloch, Darcy Carr, Darrin Pruitt, Dave Lucero, David Haddow, Debjani Das, Deborah Kapell, Debra Berg, Dena Bushman, Denise Lee, Dominique Balan, Don Olson, Eileen Rodriguez, Elisha Wilson, Ellen Gee, Ellen Lee, Elsa Huang, Elsie Estrada, Elsie Lee, Emily Lumeng-McGibbon, Emily Westheimer, Eric Peterson, Eric Rude, Eric Rude, Erich Giebelhaus, Erin Andrews, Erin Conners, Erlinda Amoroso, Eva Fabian, Fabiana Jeanty, Fabienne Laraque, Farzad Mostashari, Fatema Haque, Fazlul Chowdhury, Francesco Silverio, Gabriel Galindo, Gee Abraham, Genevieve Bergeron, Georgia Davidson, Gili Hrusa, Giselle Merizalde, Glenette Houston, Gloria Okoh, Gloria Rivera,

HaeNa Waechter, Hannah Cooper, Hannah Kubinson, Hannah
Mandel, Heather Cook, Heather Hanson, Hilary Parton, Huali
Sun, Hyacinth Bennett, Inna Katsovich, Irene Escobar, Irwin
Uhlberg, Issac Benowitz, Jacqueline Kellachan, Jane Greenko,
Janette Yung, Jasmine Abdelnabi, Jean DeWees, Jennifer
Baumgartner, Jennifer Fuld, Jennifer Hartman, Jennifer Hsieh,
Jennifer Reich, Jessica Athens, Jessica Sell, Jessie Schwartz, Jim
Miller, Joanne Casarella, Joe Conidi, Joel Ackelsberg, Jose Poy,
Joseph Real, Judy Adama, Judy Chen, Julia Latash, Karen Alroy,
Karen Phillips, Karen Schlanger, Karima Ibrahim, Kate Turner,
Kate Uranek, Katelynn Devinney, Katherine Altschaefl, Kathryn
Legaspi, Katie Bornschlegel, Kenya Murray, Keren Landman,
Kevin Guerra, Kevin Magbitang, Kim Meaning, Kristen Lee,
Kristen Moore, Lan Li, Latoya Letsome, Lauren DiBlase, Lenka
Malec, Lew Soloff, Linda Steiner-Sichel, Lisa Alleyne, Liz
Tang, Lorraine Smith, Lucretia Jones, Lucy Rhodes, Magdalena
Berger, Mansi Agarwal, Marc Paladini, Marie Bresnahan,
Marie Dorsinville, Marilyn Campbell, Marsha Radcliffe,
Martha Iwamoto, Mary Ford, Maryam Iqbal, Maura Lash,
Meetal Morjaria, Melanie Besculides, Melissa Baur, Melissa
Corcino, Melissa Ip, Melissa Marx, Meredith Eddy, Michelle
Middleton, Mike Antwi, Micheal Phillips, Miranda Moore,
Mohammed Haroon, Molly Kratz, Muhammed Iftekharuddin,
Naama Kipperman, Nadine Kela-Murphy, Nana Mensah, Nancy
Francois, Natalie Octave, Natasha McIntosh, Natasha Williams,
Nicole Acosta, Nicole Burton, Nicolette Gantt, Nimi Kadar,
Nirah Johnson, Onycha Banton, Page Keating, Pam Kellner,
Paula DelRosso, Payal Desai' Perminder Khosa, Phyllis Pope,
Prabhu Gounder, Rachel Webster, Rafael Fernandez, Rajmohan
Sunkara, Ramona Lall, Rebecca Burns, Regan Deming, Regina
Tinsdale, Renee Pouchet, Rhonda Wagner, Rich Rosselli, Rick

Heffernan, Rob Mathes, Robert Fitzhenry, Ryan Duerme, Sally
Slavinski, Sandhya Clarke, Sara Sahl, Sarah Ahmed, Scott
Harper, Sharmila Shah, Sharon Balter, Sharon Greene, Solomon
Dada, Sophia Rand, Stacey Wright, Stanley Wang, Stephanie
Ngai, Susan Anderson, Tingting Gu-Templin, Toby Keller,
Tracey Assanah-Deane, Tracy Brock-Calhoun, Trang Nguyen,
Umaima Khan, Vasudha Reddy, Verne Bethea, Vincent Law,
Viradine Dorvilus, William Lang, Yair Hazi, Yanting Huang,
Yin Lin Leung, Yuming Li, Zeenath Rehana.

ABBREVIATIONS

ABC	American Broadcasting System
AC	Assistant Commissioner
ACC	New York City Animal Care and Control
ACS	Administration for Child Services
ADA	Assistant District Attorney
AIDS	Acquired Immunodeficiency Syndrome
AMA	American Medical Association
AME	African Methodist Episcopal
AMI	American Media Incorporated
BBC	British Broadcasting Corporation
BCD	Bureau of Communicable Disease
BIN	Building identification number
BT	Bioterrorism
BTK	Acronym for Denis Rader, the bind, torture, kill serial killer
CBS	Columbia Broadcasting System
CDC	Centers for Disease Control and Prevention
CEO	Chief Economic Officer
CIDRAP	University of Minnesota Center for Infectious Disease Research and Policy
COVID-19	Illness caused by SARS-CoV-2
CPC	Central Park Conservancy
CT	Computerized axial tomography
DBCS	Deliver barcode sorting machine
D✪D	Disease Detective
DNA	Deoxyribonucleic acid
DOB	New York City Department of Buildings
DOW	BCD epidemiologist on duty
ECDC	European Center for Disease Control

ECLRS	Electronic Clinical Laboratory Reporting System
ECMO	Extra corporeal membrane oxygenation procedure
ED	Emergency department
EIA	Enzyme innuendo assay
EIS	Epidemic Intelligence Service
EMS	Emergency medical services
EHS	Division of Environmental Health Services
El	Elevated subway tracks
EPA	Environmental Protection Agency
FBI	Federal Bureau of Investigation
FDA	Food and Drug Administration
GQ1b	Anti-ganglioside antibody test for autoimmune disorders
GSU	General Surveillance Unit
H&H	Health and Hospitals, the NYC public hospital system
H1N1	Strain of influenza virus
H7N2	Strain of influenza virus
HAN	Health Alert Network
HCV	Hepatitis C virus
HIV	Human immunodeficiency virus
IBM	International Business Machines Corporation
ICS	Incident Command System
ICU	Intensive Care Unit
ILI	Influenza-like illness
K2	Type of synthetic marijuana
LD	Legionnaires' disease
LD$_{50}$	Lethal dose of a toxin poison or chemical at which 50% of the affected population die
LGBTQ	Lesbian, Gay, Bisexual, Transgender, Queer community

LP1	*Legionella pneumophila* type 1
MA	Medical assistant
MALDI-TOF	Matrix-assisted laser desorption ionization–time of flight mass spectrometry is a laboratory to identify infectious agents
MD	Meningococcal disease
MEETH	Manhattan, Eye, Ear and Throat Hospital
MERS	Middle Eastern Respiratory System virus
Mpox	Formerly called monkeypox virus
MRI	Magnetic resonance imaging
MSM	Men who have sex with men
MTA	Metropolitan Transit Authority
NAS	National Academy of Sciences
NBC	National Broadcasting Company
NPR	National Public Radio
NYC	New York City
NYSDOH	New York State Department of Health
NYPD	New York City Police Department
NYU	New York University
OCME	Office of the Chief Medical Examiner of New York
OPMC	New York State Office of Professional Medical Conduct
ORV	Oral rabies vaccine
OVS	Office of Vital Statistics
PCR	Polymerase chain reaction
PEP	Post exposure prophylaxis
PFGE	Pulsed-field gel electrophoresis
PHE	Public Health Epidemiologist
PHEng	Public Health Engineering bureau
PHL	New York City Public Health Laboratory
PHN	Public Health Nurse

PNE	Pneumonia
PPE	Personal protective equipment
PRP	Platelet rich plasma
PTC	Pain treatment center
PUI	Person under investigation for a communicable disease
RFA	Radiofrequency ablation
RIBA	Recombinant immunoblot assay
RNA	Ribonucleic acid
RSV	Respiratory Syncytial Virus
SARS	Severe acute respiratory syndrome virus that emerged in 2003
SARS-CoV-2	Severe acute respiratory syndrome coronavirus 2
SBT	Sequence-based typing
SNP	Single nucleotide polymorphism
STD / STI	Used interchangeable Sexually transmitted disease or infection
SurvEpi	Surveillance and Epidemiology emergency response group
T2	Test and Trace, system established to perform COVID-19 contact tracing
TAT	Turn-around time
TB	Tuberculosis
TF	Typhoid fever
TPOXX	Tecovirimat, a research drug for treating mpox
TVR	Trap, vaccinate, and release
USAMRIID	United States Army Medical Research Institute for Infectious Diseases
USDA	United States Department of Agriculture
USPS	United States Postal Service
Vi	Capsular polysaccharide virulence antigen
WGS	Whole genome sequencing

ENDNOTES

Chapter 2 | Guilty Fish

1 Humphrey TJ, Martin KW, and Whitehead A, "Contamination of Hands and Work Surfaces with Salmonella Enteritidis PT4 During the Preparation of Egg Dishes," *Epidemiology and Infection*, 1994; 113: 403-409.

2 "Foodborne Outbreaks, Active Multistage Outbreaks, Salmonella," CDC, accessed on August 4, 2024, https://www.cdc.gov/foodborne-outbreaks/active-investigations/index.html.

Chapter 3 | Typhoid Chicken

3 "Typhoid Fever and Paratyphoid Fever," CDC, accessed on Aug 4, 2024, https://www.cdc.gov/typhoid-fever/about.

4 "Incidence of Typhoid Fever, by Year—United States, 1920-1960," CDC, accessed on July 6, 2023, https://www.cdc.gov/mmwr/pdf/wk/mm4840.pdf

5 DiBacco, Thomas V., "When Typhoid Was Dreaded," *The Washington Post*, January 24, 1994, https://www.washingtonpost.com/archive/lifestyle/wellness/1994/01/25/when-typhoid-was-dreaded/9b2abb2d-ac05-42ae-802a-34122b16c322/.

6 Olsen SJ, Bleasdale SC, and Magnano AR, et al., "Outbreaks of Typhoid Fever in the United States, 1960-1999," *Epidemiology and Infection* 2003; 103: 13-21. DOI: 10.1017/S0950268802007598.

7 Ibid.

8 Mathieu JJ, Henning KJ, Bell E, and Frieden TR, "Typhoid Fever in New York City, 1980 Through 1990," *Archives of*

Internal Medicine, 1994; 154:1713-1718.

[9] Katz DJ, Cruz MA, Trepka MJ, Suarez JA, Fiorella PD, and Hammond RM, "An Outbreak of Typhoid Fever in Florida Associated with an Imported Frozen Fruit," *The Journal of Infectious Diseases*, 2002; 186:234–9.

[10] Leavitt JW, *Typhoid Mary*, (Boston: Beacon Press, 1996).

Chapter 4 | What Has Eight Legs and Fries?

[11] The Explorers Club, accessed on July 10, 2023, https://www.explorers.org/.

[12] Ibid.

[13] Van Huis A, Van Itterbeeck J, and Klunder H, et al. *A Edible Insects: Future Prospects for Food and Feed Security*, Food and Agriculture Organization of the United Nations, Rome, 2013.

[14] Ibid.

[15] Eplett L, "Metamorphosis: How to Change Our Perception of Eating Insects," accessed on July 12, 2023, https://www.laylaeplett.com/culinary-arts/blog-post-title-one-xbwge.

[16] NBC News, "Tarantula Shoots Sharp Hairs Into Owners Eyes," January 1, 2010, accessed on July 21, 2023, https://www.nbcnews.com/health/health-news/tarantula-shoots-sharp-hairs-owner-s-eye-flna1c9440850.

Chapter 5 | First Do No Hepatitis

[17] Balter S, Stark JH, Kennedy J, Bornschlegel K, and Kothy K, "Estimating the Prevalence of Hepatitis C infection in New York City Using Surveillance Data," *Epidemiology and Infection.*. 2014; 142: 262–269. .doi: 10.1017/S0950268813000952.

[18] Petruzziello A, Marigliano S, Loquercio G, Cozzolino A, and Cacciapuoti C, "Global Epidemiology of Hepatitis C virus Infection: An Update of the Distribution and Circulation of

Hepatitis C Virus Genotype, *World Journal of Gastroenterology*, 2016; 22(34): 7824-7840. DOI: 10.3748/wjg.v22.i34.7824.

[19] Esteban JI, Gomez J, and Martell M, et al., "Transmission of Hepatitis C Virus by a Cardiac Surgeon, *The New England Journal of Medicine*, 1996; 334: 555-560.

[20] Cody SH, Naiman OV, and Garfein RS, "Hepatitis C Virus Transmission from an Anesthesiologist to a Patient," *Archives of Internal Medicine*, 2003; 162: 345-350.

[21] "Prescription Value & Pricing," drug price list, Pfizer.com, accessed on April 4, 2024, https://www.pfizer.com/about/programs-policies/prescription-value-and-pricing.

[22] Food and Drug Administration, "Selection of the Appropriate Package Type Terms and Recommendations for Labeling Injectable Medical Products Packaged in Multiple-Dose, Single-Dose, and Single-Patient-Use Containers for Human Use Guidance for Industry," accessed on July 21, 2023, https://www.fda.gov/media/117883/download.

[23] Plott RT, Wagner RF, and Tyring SK, "Iatrogenic Contamination of Multidose Vials in Simulated Use, *Archives of Dermatology*, 1990; 126: 1441-1444.

[24] Trasancos CC, Kainer MA, Desmond PV, and Kell H, "Investigation of Potential Iatrogenic Transmission of Hepatitis C in Victoria, Australia," *Australian and New Zealand Journal of Public Health*, 2001; 25(3): 241-244.

[25] Massari M, Petrosillo N, and Ippolito G et al., "Transmission of Hepatitis C Virus in a Gynecological Surgery Setting," *Journal of Clinical Microbiology*. 2001; 39 (8): 2860–2863. DOI: 10.1128/JCM.39.8.2860–2863.

[26] Campanile C. "State OKs Scandal Docs," *The New York Post*, April 2, 2007. Accessed on June 7, 2024, from https://nypost.com/2007/04/02/state-oks-scandal-docs/

Chapter 6 | Death by Post

[27] Meselson M, Guillemin J, and Hugh-Jones M, et al., "The Sverdlovsk Anthrax Outbreak of 1979," *Science*, 1994; 266: 1202-1208.

[28] Beecher DJ, "Forensic Application of Microbiological Culture Analysis To Identify Mail Intentionally Contaminated with *Bacillus Anthracis* Spores," *Applied and Environmental Microbiology*, 2006; 72(8): 5304-5310. doi:10.1128/AEM.00940-06.

[29] Kournikakis B, Armour SJ, Boulet CA, Spence M, and Parsons B, "Risk Assessment of Anthrax Letters," Defense Research Establishment Suffield Technical Report, DRES, September 2001, TR-2001-048.

[30] Freed D. "The Wrong Man." *The Atlantic*, May 2010. Accessed on April 2, 2024, from https://www.theatlantic.com/magazine/archive/2010/05/the-wrong-man/308019/

[31] Ibid

[32] United States Department of Justice. Amerithrax Investigative Summary. Accessed on April 1, 2024, from https://www.justice.gov/archive/amerithrax/docs/amx-investigative-summary.pdf

[33] National Academy of Sciences, "Review of the Scientific Approaches Used During the FBI's Investigation of the 2001 Anthrax Letters," National Academy of Sciences Press, Washington, D.C., 2011, https://nap.nationalacademies.org/catalog/13098/review-of-the-scientific-approaches-used-during-the-fbis-investigation-of-the-2001-anthrax-letters.

Chapter 7 | Pain From a Pain Clinic

[34] Institute of Medicine, *Relieving Pain in America: A Blueprint for Transforming Prevention, Care, Education, and Research*, 2011,

Washington, DC: The National Academies Press.

[35] Prescient and Strategic Intelligence, *Chronic Pain Treatment Market Size & Share Analysis—Trends, Drivers, Competitive Landscape, and Forecasts (2024–2030)*, accessed on August 6, 2024, https://www.psmarketresearch.com/market-analysis/chronic-pain-treatment-market.

[36] Niewijk G, "Ancient Analgesics: A Brief History of Opioids," *Yale Scientific Magazine*, accessed on March 13, 2024, https://www.yalescientic.org/author/graceniewijk/.

[37] Sabatowski R, Schäfer D, Kasper SM, Brunsch H, and Radbruch L, "Pain Treatment: A Historical Overview," *Current Pharmaceutical Design*, 2004; 10: 701-716.

[38] Ibid.

[39] CDC. "Bacterial Meningitis After Intrapartum Spinal Anesthesia—New York and Ohio, 2008–2009." *MMWR.* 2010; 59(3): 65-67.

[40] Comstock RD, Melanie S, and Fox JL, et al., "A Large Nosocomial Outbreak of Hepatitis C and Hepatitis B Among Patients Receiving Pain Remediation Treatments," *Infection Control and Hospital Epidemiology*, 2004; 25: 576-583.

[41] Cohen AL, Ridpath A, and Noble-Wang J, et al., "Outbreak of Serratia Marcescens Bloodstream and Central Nervous System Infections After Interventional Pain Management Procedures," *Clinical Journal of Pain*, 2008; 24: 374-380.

[42] Matter F and Gastmeir P, "Bacterial Contamination of Multiple-Dose Vials: A Prevalence Study," *American Journal of Infection Control*, 2004; 32(1): 12-16.

[43] Buffet-Bataillon S, Rabier V, and Betermieux P, et al., "Outbreak of Serratia Marcescens in a Neonatal Intensive Care Unit: Contaminated Unmedicated Liquid Soap and Risk Factors," *Journal of Hospital Infection*, 2009; 7: 17-22. doi:10.1016/j.

jhin.2009.01.010.

44 CDC. "Multistate Outbreak of Fungal Infection Associated with Injection of Methylprednisolone Acetate Solution from a Single Compounding Pharmacy — United States, 2012." *MMWR.* 2012; 61(41);839-842. Accessed on November 8, 2024, from https://www.cdc.gov/mmwr/preview/mmwrhtml/mm6141a4.htm

45 FDA, "New England Compounding Center Pharmacist Sentenced for Role in Nationwide Fungal Meningitis Outbreak," January 31, 2018, https://www.fda.gov/inspections-compliance-enforcement-and-criminal-investigations/press-releases/january-31-2018-new-england-compounding-center-pharmacist-sentenced-role-nationwide-fungal.

46 Scutti S, "More Men, Younger Americans Having Joint Replacement Surgery," *CNN Health*, March 6, 2018, August 7, 2024, https://www.cnn.com/2018/03/06/health/hip-knee-replacement-surgeries-earlier-study/index.html.

47 Reports and Insights, *Interventional Pain Management Market*, Accessed on March 16, 2024, https://www.reportsandinsights.com/report/interventional-pain-management-market.

Chapter 8 | On the Trail of a Serial Killer

48 County Court of Suffolk County, "The People of the State of New York against Rex A. Heuermann. CPL 530.40 Bail Application. Accessed on November 9, 2024 from https://int.nyt.com/data/documenttools/lti-bail-application-form-2023-7-14-23-final-1-redacted-1/6ffd72d59b87aa51/full.pdf

49 Shapiro A. "Police Use DNA to Track Suspects Through Family." NPR *All Things Considered,* December 12, 2007. Accessed on November 9, 2024 from https://www.npr.org/2007/12/12/17130501/

police-use-dna-to-track-suspects-through-family

[50] Krause G, Blackmore C, and Wiersma S, et al., "Marijuana Use and Social Networks in a Community Outbreak of Meningococcal Disease," *Southern Medical Journal*, 2001; 94: 482-485.

[51] Cohen C, Singh E, and Wu HM, et al., "Increased Incidence of Meningococcal Disease in HIV-Infected Associated with an Increased Case Fatality Rate," *AIDS*, 2010: 24: 1351-1360.

[52] Miller L, Arakaki L, and Ramautar A, et al., "Elevated Risk for Invasive Meningococcal Disease Among Persons With HIV," *Annals of Internal Medicine*, 2014; 160: 30-37. doi: 10.7326/0003-4819-160-1-201401070-00731.

[53] NYC Department of Health and Mental Hygiene, "Update: Meningococcal Vaccine Recommendations for HIV-Infected Men Who Have Sex With Men," Health Alert 28, October 4, 2012.

[54] NYC Department of Health and Mental Hygiene, "Update: Meningococcal Vaccine Recommendations for HIV-Infected Men Who Have Sex With Men, Two Cases Reported in the Past Five Weeks," Health Alert 36, November 29, 2012.

[55] Bazan JA, Peterson AS, and Kirkcaldy RA, et al. Increase in *Neisseria Meningitidis*–Associated Urethritis Among Men at Two Sentinel Clinics—Columbus, Ohio, and Oakland County, Michigan, 2015," *MMWR*. 2017; 65(21): 550-552. doi:10.15585/mmwr.mm6521a5.

[56] Rodriguez EI, Tzeng YL, and Stephens DS, "Continuing Genomic Evolution of the *Neisseria Meningitidis* cc11.2 urethritis clade, NmUC: A Narrative Review," *Microbial Genetics*, 2023; 9: 001113. 2023;9:001113 DOI 10.1099/mgen.0.001113.

[57] Bazan JA, Stephens DS, and Turner Norris A, "Emergence

of a Novel Urogenital-Tropic *Neisseria Meningitidis*," *Current Opinion Infectious Disease*, 2021; 34: 34-39. doi:10.1097/QCO.0000000000000697.

[58] Faur YC, Weisburd MH, and Wilson ME, "Isolation of *Neisseria Meningitidis* from the Genitourinary Tract and Anal Canal," *Journal of Clinical Microbiology*, 1975; 2: 178-182.

[59] Kretz CB, Bergeron B, and Aldrich M, et al., "Neonatal Conjunctivitis Caused by *Neisseria Meningitidis* US Urethritis Clade, New York, August 2017," *Emerging Infectious Diseases*, 2019; 25: 972-976.

[60] Mandal S, Wu HM, and MacNeil JR, et al., "Prolonged University Outbreak of Meningococcal Disease Associated With a Serogroup B Strain Rarely Seen in the United States," *Clinical Infectious Diseases*, 2013; 57: 344-348.

[61] Soeters HM, McNamara LA, and Blain AE, et al., "University-Based Outbreaks of Meningococcal Disease Caused by Serogroup B, United States, 2013–2018" *Emerging Infectious Diseases*, 2019; 25: 434-440.

[62] CDC, "Prevention and Control of *Haemophilus Influenzae* Type B Disease," *MMWR*, 2014; 63: 1-20.

[63] CDC HAN, "Increase in Invasive Serogroup Y Meningococcal Disease in the United States," March 28, 2024, https://emergency.cdc.gov/han/2024/han00505.asp.

Chapter 9 | Bandits in the Park

[64] Pasteur Foundation, *Institut Pasteur and US Historic Relations*, October 16, 2010, https://pasteurfoundation.org/about/history/

[65] Fitzsimmons EG. "Robert F. Kennedy Jr. Admits He Left a Dead Bear in Central Park," *The New York Times*, August 4, 2024. Accessed on November 10, 2024 from https://www.

nytimes.com/2024/08/04/us/politics/robert-f-kennedy-jr-
bear-central-park.html

Chapter 10 | Dying to Be Beautiful

[66] Market Watch, "$220+ Billion Non-Invasive Aesthetic Treatment Market by Procedure, Injectables, Skin Rejuvenation, Gender, End User, Country and Company Analysis—Global Forecast to 2032," accessed on May 23, 2024, https://www.marketwatch. com/press-release/220-billion-non-invasive-aesthetic-treat-ment-market-by-procedure-injectables-skin-rejuvena-tion-gender-end-user-country-and-company-analysis-glob-al-forecast-to-2032-researchandmarkets-com-20abc41b.

[67] IBIS World, "Plastic Surgeons in the US—Market Research Report," January 23, 2024, https://www.ibisworld.com/ united-states/market-research-reports/?entid=4157.

[68] Wilson J, "Cosmetic Surgery Is On The Rise With Technology And Hollywood Is At The Center Of It," *Forbes.* January 18, 2023, https://www.forbes.com/sites/joshwilson/2023/01/18/ cosmetic-surgery-is-on-the-rise-with-technology-and-hol-lywood-is-at-the-centre-of-it/?sh=274ce0441d91.

[69] Cacciatore B. "Celebrity Plastic Surgery: 31 Stars Who Have Admitted to 'Getting Work Done,'" *Glamour,* October 8, 2024. Accessed on November 11, 2024 from https://www.glamour. com/gallery/celebrity-plastic-surgery-and-injectables

[70] Toy BR and Frank PJ, "Outbreak of Mycobacterium Abscessus Infection After Soft Tissue Augmentation," *Dermatologic Surgery,* 2003: 29: 971-973.

[71] District Attorney for Queens County, Press Release, "Queens Spa Owner Pleads Guilty to Unlawfully Practicing Medicine and Seriously Injuring Client," May 30, 2012, https://www.yumpu.com/en/document/read/25623592/

for-immediate-release-contact-queens-county-district-attorney.

[72] Ibid.

[73] United States Department of Justice, Southern District of New York. Press Release: "Manhattan US Attorney Charges Bronx Woman with Illegal Administration of Liquid Silicone Injections Through Underground Business, January 14, 2011." Accessed on July 23, 2024 from https://www.justice.gov/archive/usao/nys/pressreleases/January11/castillowhalesca-complaintpr.pdf

[74] District Attorney, Bronx County, NY. "Bronx Woman Sentenced to 4-8 Years in Prison for Death of Woman she Injected with Silicone, February 22, 2024." Accessed on July 24, 2024 from https://www.bronxda.nyc.gov/downloads/pdf/pr/2024/15-2024%20Whalesca-Castillo-sentenced-manslaughter.pdf

[75] Carlin D, "Bronx Woman Sentenced to Prison for Deadly Unlicensed Cosmetic Surgery," *CBS News*, February 22, 2024, https://www.cbsnews.com/newyork/news/whalesca-castillo-deadly-unlicensed-cosmetic-surgery-sentencing.

[76] Smith SW, Graber NM, Johnson RC, Barr JR, Hoffman RS, and Nelson LS, "Multisystem Organ Failure After Large Volume Injection of Castor Oil," *Annals of Plastic Surgery*, 2009, 62: 12-14.

[77] Associated Press, "Black Madam Gets 10 Years After Buttocks-Enhancement Death," June 15, 2011, https://whyy.org/articles/black-madam-gets-10-years-after-buttocks-enhancement-death/.

[78] Harris P and Davis R, "Cosmetic Surgery in American Hotel Leads to Death of British Woman," *The Guardian*, February 9, 2011, https://www.theguardian.com/lifeandstyle/2011/feb/09/cosmetic-surgery-british-woman.

Chapter 11 | The Mummy of Queens

[79] "Smallpox Extinction—A Note of Caution," The New Scientist, originally published July 1, 1976, republished November 16, 2006, https://www.newscientist.com/article/dn10544-smallpox-extinction-a-note-of-caution/.

[80] Ibid.

[81] Edwards LF, *Cincinnati's Old Cunny, A Notorious Purveyor of Human Flesh*, Public Library of Fort Wayne and Allen County, 1955, The Gutenberg Book Project, accessed on April 24, 2024, fromhttps://www.gutenberg.org/files/65856/65856-h/65856-h.htm.

[82] Wolff HL and Croon JJ, "The Survival of Smallpox (Variola Minor) in Natural Circumstances," *Bulletin of the World Health Organization*, 1968; 38: 492-493.

[83] Alix B, "Smallpox Scab Seized from Richmond Museum," *The Richmond Times-Dispatch*, May 19, 2011, https://richmond.com/smallpox-scab-seized-from-richmond-museum/article_f77dadc2-6f04-5ad8-8281-224e1b4dd473.html.

[84] McCollum AM, Yu L, and Wilkins K, et al., "Poxvirus Viability and Signatures in Historical Relics," *Emerging Infectious Diseases*, 2014; 20: 177-184. DOI: http://dx.doi.org/10.3201/eid2002.131098.

[85] Biagini P, Theves C, Bararesque P, "Variola Virus in a 300-Year Old Siberian Mummy," *The New England Journal of Medicine*, 2012; 367: 2057-2059.

[86] Warnasch S, "Newark's Iron Coffins and Mummies," *Iron Coffin Mummy*, accessed on April 19, 2024, https://ironcoffin-mummy.com.

[87] Vittek S, "Newark's Mummies Raise Many Grave Questions," *New Jersey Monthly*, May 5, 2017, https://ironcoffinmummy.com/new-jersey-monthly-newarks-mummies-raise-many-

grave-questions/.

[88] US Census, "1850 Census: The Seventh Census of the United States," accessed on April 12, 2024, https://www.census.gov/library/publications/1853/dec/1850a.html.

[89] US Census, "Decennial Census Official Publications," accessed on April 12, 2024, https://www.census.gov/programs-surveys/decennial-census/decade/decennial-publications.1830.html.

[90] US Census, "Decennial Census Official Publications," https://www.census.gov/programs-surveys/decennial-census/decade/decennial-publications.1840.html#list-tab-799609106.

[91] Williams L, "Martha Peterson of Newtown: The Woman in the Iron Coffin," November 23, 2019, https://margoleewilliamsbooks.com/2019/11/23/martha-peterson-of-newtown-the-woman-in-the-iron-coffin/.

[92] Leavitt JW, "Be Safe, Be Sure, New York's Experience with Smallpox," *Hives of Sickness,* New Brunswick, NJ: Rutgers University Press, 1995.

[93] Quinn RL, Warnasch SC, Watson M, et al. "Biogeochemical evidence for residence, diet, and health of the Woman in the Iron Coffin (Queens, New York City)." *Int. J. Osteoarchaeol.,* 2020; 30:225-235.

[94] *Secrets of the Dead*, S16, Ep 5. "The Woman in the Iron Coffin," original air date October 3, 2018, https://www.pbs.org/wnet/secrets/woman-in-the-iron-coffin-about-the-film/3923/.

[95] Redmond C, "Mystery Of Shockingly Well-Preserved Mummy Found in New York City Finally Solved," *All That's Interesting,* October 3, 2018, accessed on April 24, 2024, https://allthatsinteresting.com/martha-peterson-iron-coffin.

Chapter 12 | South Bronx in the Crosshairs Again

[96] National Weather Service, "Average Monthly and Annual

Temperatures," accessed on May 5, 2024, https://www.weather.gov/media/okx/Climate/CentralPark/monthlyannualtemp.pdf.

[97] World Health Organization, "Ebola, West Africa, March 2014-2016," accessed on August 10, 2024, https://www.who.int/emergencies/situations/ebola-outbreak-2014-2016-West-Africa.

[98] Osterholm MT, Chin TDY, and Osborne DO, et al., "A 1957 Outbreak of Legionnaires' Disease Associated with a Meat Packing Plant," *American Journal of Epidemiology*, 1983; 117: 60-67.

[99] "Cooling Towers Market Size, Share & Industry Analysis, By Type (Wet, Dry, and Hybrid)," *Fortune Business Insights*, July 22, 2024, https://www.fortunebusinessinsights.com/enquiry/request-sample-pdf/102747.

[100] "Electronic Registration Systems for Cooling Towers," Urban Sustainability Systems Network, accessed on August 11, 2024, https://www.usdn.org/uploads/cms/documents/deliverable_3_cooling_towers_technical_paper_lt_0120_digital.pdf.

[101] "Cooling Tower Inspection Results," NYC Department of Health and Mental Hygiene, accessed on August 11, 2024, https://www.nyc.gov/site/doh/business/permits-and-licenses/cooling-towers-inspection-results.page.

[102] García-Fulgueiras A, Navarro C, and Fenoll D, et al., "Legionnaires' Disease Outbreak in Murcia, Spain," *Emerging Infectious Diseases*, 2003; 9:915-921.

[103] Greig JE, Carnie JA, and Tallis GF, et al., "An Outbreak of Legionnaires' Disease at the Melbourne Aquarium, April 2000: Investigation and Case-Control Studies," *Medical Journal of Australia*, 2004; 180: 566-572.

[104] Bennett E, Ashton M, and Calverts N, et al., "Barrow-in-Furness:

A Large Community Legionellosis Outbreak in the UK," *Epidemiology and Infection*, 2014; 142: 1763-1777. doi:10.1017/S0950268813002483.

[105] George F, Shivaji T, and Pinto C, et al., "A Large Outbreak of Legionnaires' Disease in an Industrial Town in Portugal," *Revista Portugesa de Saude Publica*, 2016; 34: 199-208, http://dx.doi.org/10.1016/j.rpsp.2016.10.001.

Chapter 13 | Muerto Vivero

[106] Sejvar J, Bancroft E, and Winthrop K, et al. Leptospirosis, "Eco-Challenge Athletes, Malaysian Borneo, 2000" *Emerging Infectious Diseases*, 2003;9: 702-707.

[107] Stern EJ, Galloway R, and Shadowy SV, et al., "Outbreak of Leptospirosis Among Adventure Race Participants in Florida, 2005," *Clinical Infectious Diseases*, 2010; 50: 843-849. DOI: 10.1086/650578.

Chapter 14 | It Was Only a Question of When

[108] Bellafante G, "The Mayor New Yorkers Love to Hate," *The New York Times*, December 23, 2021, https://www.nytimes.com/2021/12/23/nyregion/bill-de-blasio-mayor-nyc.html.

[109] Ibid.

[110] Ibid.

[111] Reuters, "Chinese Authorities Say Viral Pneumonia is Not SARS, MERS, or Bird Flu," accessed on August 12, 2024, https://sg.news.yahoo.com/chinese-authorities-viral-pneumonia-outbreak-150344412.html.

[112] CDC HAN, "Update and Interim Guidance on Outbreak of 2019 Novel Coronavirus (2019-nCoV) in Wuhan, China," accessed on June 27, 2024, https://archive.cdc.gov/#/details?q=https://emergency.cdc.gov/han/han00426.

asp&start=0&rows=10&url=https://emergency.cdc.gov/han/han00426.asp.

[113] Rothe C, Schunk M, and Sothmann, et al., "Letter: Transmission of 2019-nCoV Infection from an Asymptomatic Contact in Germany," *The New England Journal of Medicine*, 2020; 382: 970-72. DOI: 10.1056/NEJMc2001468.

[114] Huang C, Wang Y, and Li X, et al., "Clinical Features of Patients Infected with 2019 Novel Coronavirus in Wuhan, China," *Lancet*, 2020; 395:497-506. https://doi.org/10.1016/.

[115] Smith GB, "In Note to Fauci, Top City Doctor Takes Shot at de Blasio's COVID-19 Contact Tracing Program," *The City*, January 28, 2021, https://www.thecity.nyc/2021/01/28/fauci-vaccinations-de-blasios-nyc-covid-contact-tracing/.

[116] "COVID-19: Data," NYC DOHMH's *Long-Term Trends*, accessed on July 18. 2024, https://www.nyc.gov/site/doh/covid/covid-19-data-totals.page.

[117] "Revenue of Laboratory Corporation of America," 103 Statista, accessed on July 17, 2024, https://www.statista.com/statistics/859710/labcorp-revenue/.

[118] "Quest Diagnostics Gross Profits 2010-2014," Macrotrends, accessed on July 17, 2024, https://www.macrotrends.net/stocks/charts/DGX/quest-diagnostics/gross-profit.

[119] "Historical Price Lookup," Labcorp, accessed on July 17, 2024, https://ir.labcorp.com/financials/historical-price-lookup.

[120] "Historical Price Lookup," Quest Diagnostics, accessed on July 17, 2024, https://ir.questdiagnostics.com/stock-info/historical-price-lookup/default.aspx.

[121] Varma J, Thamkittikasem J, and Whittemore K, et al., "COVID-19 Infections Among Students and Staff in New York City Public Schools," *Pediatrics*, 2021; 147: 1-8. DOI: https://doi.org/10.1542/peds.2021-050605.

[122] McMichael TM, Clark S, and Pogojans S, et al., "COVID-19 in a Long-Term Care Facility— ing County, Washington, February 27–March 9, 2020," *MMWR*, 2020; 69: 339-342.

[123] Liu W, Chen J, and Xiang R, et al., "Letter to the Editor: Detection of Covid-19 in Children in Early January 2020 in Wuhan, China," *The New England Journal of Medicine*, 2020; 382; 1370-1372. DOI: 10.1056/NEJMc2003717.

[124] Hernandez MM, Gonzalez-Reiche AS, and Alshammary A, et al., "Molecular Evidence of SARS-CoV-2 in New York Before the First Pandemic Wave," *Nature Communications*, 2021; 1-8. https://doi.org/10.1038/s41467-021-23688-7.

[125] "COVID-19: Data," NYC DOHMH's *Latest Data*, accessed on August 12. 2024, https://www.nyc.gov/site/doh/covid/covid-19-data.page#daily.

Chapter 15 | Not All Mystery Diseases Are Infectious

[126] Blum D, *The Poisoner's Handbook*, New York: Penguin Press, 2010.

[127] Schottelkotte S, "Grim Milestone: 20 Years on Death Row," *The Ledger*, March 5, 2011, https://www.theledger.com/story/news/2011/03/05/grim-milestone-20-years-on/8051384007/.

[128] Deak M, "NJ Court Upholds Murder Conviction of Monroe Chemist Who Poisoned Her Husband, *My Central Jersey*, June 26, 2021, https://www.mycentraljersey.com/story/news/local/courts/2021/06/26/nj-court-upholds-murder-conviction-chemist-who-poisoned-her-husband/5345282001/.

[129] ChatGPT4, accessed on June 25, 2024, https://chatgpt.com/.

Chapter 16 | Did the Commissioner Diddle While Rectums Burned?

[130] Melski J, Reed K, and Stratton E, et al., "Multistate Outbreak

of Monkeypox—Illinois, Indiana, and Wisconsin, 2003," *MMWR*, 2003: 52: 537-540.

[131] Reed KD, Melski JW, and Graham MB, et al., "The Detection of Monkeypox in Humans in the Western Hemisphere," *The New England Journal of Medicine*, 2004; 350: 342-350.

[132] Eisenberg A, "New City Health Commissioner Has History of Leadership Issues in Previous Role," *Politico*, March 21, 2022, https://www.politico.com/news/2022/03/21/new-city-health-commissioner-has-history-of-leadership-issues-in-previous-role-00018527.

[133] "Monkeypox Cases Reported in UK and Portugal," European Centre for Disease Control and Prevention's press release, May 19, 2022, https://www.ecdc.europa.eu/en/news-events/monkeypox-cases-reported-uk-and-portugal.

[134] "Show Your Pride and Stay Healthy, Says Health Department," NYC DOHMH's press release, accessed on August 13, 2024, https://www.nyc.gov/site/doh/about/press/pr2022/show-your-pride-and-stay-healthy-says-health-department.page.

[135] Ogonie D, Izibewule JH, and Ogunleye A, et al., "The 2017 Human Monkeypox Outbreak in Nigeria—Report of Outbreak Experience and Response in the Niger Delta University Teaching Hospital, Bayelsa State, Nigeria," *PLOS One*, 2019, https://doi.org/10.1371/journal.pone.0214229; 14: e0214229.

[136] CDC HAN, "Monkeypox Virus Infection in the United States and Other Non-endemic Countries—2022," CDCHAN-00466, May 20, 2022, accessed on July 24, 2024, https://emergency.cdc.gov/han/2022/han00466.asp.

[137] Soucheray S, "Experts Aim to Thread Needle on Monkeypox Messaging to MSM," Center for Infectious Disease Research and Policy (CIDRAP), June 9, 2022, https://www.cidrap.umn.edu/

experts-aim-thread-needle-monkeypox-messaging-msm.

[138] Sandman P, "Avoiding Stigmatization Shouldn't Be the Top Priority in Monkeypox Risk Communication," two emails shared with CIDRAP and posted on The Peter Sandman Risk Communication website, accessed on July 11, 2024, https://www.psandman.com/articles/Monkeypox1.htm.

[139] Westbrook E, "Second Day of Long Lines for Monkeypox Vaccine at Chelsea Sexual Health Clinic," *CBS News New York*, June 24, 2022, https://www.cbsnews.com/newyork/news/second-day-of-long-lines-for-monkeypox-vaccine-at-chelsea-sexual-health-clinic/.

[140] "Interview with Kavita Patel: Making Sense of Monkeypox," MSNBC's *The Sunday Show*, July 3, 2022, https://www.facebook.com/msnbc/videos/dr-kavita-patel-making-sense-of-monkeypox/1190530618186967/.

[141] "NYC Health Department on Monkeypox Vaccination Strategy and Prioritization of First Doses," NYC DOHMH's press release, July 15, 2022, https://www.nyc.gov/site/doh/about/press/pr2022/monkeypox-vaccination-prioritization-first-doses.page.

[142] Goldstein J, "Debate Over Monkeypox Messaging Divides N.Y.C. Health Department," *The New York Times*, July 18, 2022, https://www.nytimes.com/2022/07/18/nyregion/nyc-monkeypox-health-department-information-inaccurate.html.

[143] Thomas N, "NYC Monkeypox Numbers Are 'Definitively' Not the Full Picture, Health Official Says," *CNN*, July 21, 2022, https://www.cnn.com/2022/07/19/health/nyc-health-commissioner-monkeypox/index.html.

[144] Deputy NP, Decker J, and Chard AN, et al., "Vaccine Effectiveness of JYNNEOS Against Mpox Disease in the

United States," *The New England Journal of Medicine*, 2023; 388: 2434-2444. DOI: 10.1056/NEJMoa2215201.

145 Op. cit. Thomas.

146 Ryan B, "You Are Being Misled About Monkeypox, *Washington Post*, July 18, 2022, https://www.washingtonpost.com/opinions/2022/07/18/monkeypox-gay-men-deserve-unvarnished-truth/.

147 Ryan B, "Opinion: Gay Men Can Fight Monkeypox Ourselves—By Changing How We Have Sex," *The Washington Post*, August 11, 2022, https://www.washingtonpost.com/opinions/2022/08/11/monkeypox-gay-sex-guidelines/.

148 King MS, "Monkeypox is a Gay Thing. We Must Say It," *POZ*, July 21, 2022, accessed https://www.poz.com/blog/monkeypox-gay-thing-must-say#search-query=monkeypox.

149 Downs J, "Gay Men Need a Specific Warning About Monkeypox," *The Atlantic*, May 28, 2022, https://www.theatlantic.com/ideas/archive/2022/05/monkeypox-outbreak-spread-gay-bi-sexual-men/643122/.

150 *Doctor with a Badge,* blog comments, accessed on August 2, 2024, https://doctor-with-a-badge.webnode.page/support/.

151 Ward T, Christie R, Paton RS, Chumming F, and Overton CE, "Transmission Dynamics of Monkeypox in the United Kingdom: Contact Tracing Study," *British Medical Journal*, 2022; 379: e073153. doi: 10.1136/bmj-2022-073153.

152 Shapiro A, "White House 'Cautiously Optimistic' on Monkeypox," NPR *All Things Considered* interview with Dr. Demetre Daskalakis, September 28, 2022.

Epilogue | The Future of Public Health

153 Lewis C. "NYC health commissioner to step down Friday, months earlier than expected." *The Gothamist*, October 15,

2024. Accessed on October 16, 2024 from https://gothamist.com/news/nyc-health-commissioner-to-step-down-friday-months-earlier-than-expected

INDEX

A

Ackelsberg, Joel, 82, 251

Acquired Immunodeficiency
Syndrome (AIDS), 133,
154, 206, 324, 341

Adams, Mayor, 342

Administration for Child
Services (ACS), 298, 302

Advanced Organic Chemistry,
5

African Methodist Episcopal
(AME), 93-96, 186, 190

Al Qaeda attack, 77

Aldrich M, 360n59

Alix B, 363n83

Ambrosi, Corinne, 189

Amebiasis, 8

American Broadcasting
System (ABC), 78

American Media Incorporated
(AMI), 82

American Medical Association
(AMA), 308

Amoroso, Elrinda, 242

Angiocatheter, 65, 68-69

Animal Care and Control
(ACC), 155, 160, 164

Arakaki L, 359n52

Arizona, 93, 135, 141, 253

Armour SJ, 356n29

Ashcroft, John, 93

Ashton M, 365n104

Aspirin, 100, 298

Assistant Commissioner (AC),
13, 37, 76, 219, 250, 298,
302

Assistant District Attorney
(ADA), 181-182

Attack Rates, 52-53

Australia, 60, 70, 213, 253,
313

Ayala, Lesbia, 183

Italy, 188, 264, 267, 313

Ivins, Bruce, 94-95, 97

J

James, Letitia, 245

Japan, 135, 252-253, 264

Jenner, Edward, 153, 187

Johnson RC, 362n76

Jones, Lucretia, 110, 204

K

K. pneumoniae, 104

Kainer MA, 355n24

Kasper SM, 357n37

Kass, Dan, 219, 223, 226, 249

Katsovich, Inna, 110

Katz DJ, 354n9

Kell H, 355n24

Kennedy J, 354n17

Kennedy, Robert F., Jr., 169

King MS, 371n148

Kirkcaldy RA, 359n55

Klebsiella pneumonia, 104, 109

Klunder H, 354n13

Korea, 96, 253, 267

Kornblum, John, 112

Kothy K, 354n17

Kournikakis B, 356n29

Kratz, Molly, 139

Krause G, 359n50

Kretz CB, 360n59

L

Layton, Marci, 37, 85, 219, 273, 280, 292, 333

Leavitt JW, 354n10, 364n92

Lee, Ellen, 324

Lee, Lillian, 112

Legionella, 201-207, 210, 212-219, 227-231, 249, 251

Legionella, Legionella pneumophila (Lp), 207

Legionella pneumophila, 202, 207

Legionella Pneumophila Type 1 (LP1), 207, 218, 226, 228, 230

Legionella species, 202

Matrix-Assisted Laser
  Desorption
  Ionization-Time of Flight
  Mass Spectrometry
  (MALDI-TOF), 301
Matter F, 357n42
McCollum AM, 363n84
McDonald, Audra, 155
McMichael TM, 368n122
McNamara LA, 360n61
MD risk, 138
Medical Assistant (MA),
  19-20, 60, 66-68, 108
Meister, Joseph, 153
Melanie S, 357n40
Melski J, 368n130
Melski JW, 369n131
Men Who Have Sex with
  Men (MSM), 139-141,
  200, 313-318, 322,
  325-328, 334-335
Meningitis, 31, 102, 115-121,
  135-138, 145, 235, 241

Meningococcal Disease (MD),
  115-138, 140-147, 199, 274
Meningococcal disease MD,
  symptoms of, 129
Meningococcemia, 120, 125,
  135-136
MERS, 198, 248, 257, 274
Meselson M, 356n27
Metropolitan Transit
  Authority (MTA), 86-87,
  272
microorganisms, 8
Midazolam, 64-65, 69, 71
Middle Eastern Respiratory
  Syndrome (MERS), 198,
  248, 257, 274
Miller Fisher Syndrome,
  296-297
Miller, Judith, 83
Miller, Laura, 132, 359n52
Moraxella catarrhalis, 119
Mostashari, Farzad, 254
Mullins, Joe, 195
Multi-dose vials, 66, 70,

ABOUT THE AUTHOR

DON WEISS was born in the Bronx and composed his first story at the age of six while sitting on the stoop of his Inwood apartment. It was an illustrated story about the misadventures of a neighborhood boy named Andy. He attended a small liberal arts college in Pennsylvania and embarked on a career as a chemist before switching to medicine. He practiced urban pediatrics in New York City and the Midwest for seven years and then entered the field of public health. He was an infectious disease epidemiologist for the New York City Department of Health for 23 years. He has written four novels, three of which are public health mysteries, and served as a script and set consultant for the major motion picture, *Contagion*. Don currently is an assistant women's basketball coach and adjunct professor of public health..

Website: https://doctor-with-a-badge.webnode.page/

www.ingramcontent.com/pod-product-compliance
Lightning Source LLC
Chambersburg PA
CBHW062112020426
42335CB00013B/939